Cambridge Elements ≡

Elements in Genetics in Epilepsy
edited by
Annapurna H. Poduri
Boston Children's Hospital, Harvard Medical School
Alfred L. George, Jr.
Northwestern University Feinberg School of Medicine
Erin L. Heinzen
University of North Carolina, Chapel Hill
Daniel Lowenstein
University of California, San Francisco
Sara James
Journalist and author

HOW WE GOT TO WHERE WE'RE GOING

Annapurna H. Poduri

Boston Children's Hospital, Harvard Medical School

Alfred L. George, Jr.

Northwestern University Feinberg School of Medicine

Erin L. Heinzen

University of North Carolina, Chapel Hill

Daniel Lowenstein

University of California, San Francisco

Sara James

Journalist and author

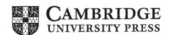

CAMBRIDGE
UNIVERSITY PRESS

CAMBRIDGE
UNIVERSITY PRESS

University Printing House, Cambridge CB2 8BS, United Kingdom

One Liberty Plaza, 20th Floor, New York, NY 10006, USA

477 Williamstown Road, Port Melbourne, VIC 3207, Australia

314–321, 3rd Floor, Plot 3, Splendor Forum, Jasola District Centre, New Delhi – 110025, India

103 Penang Road, #05–06/07, Visioncrest Commercial, Singapore 238467

Cambridge University Press is part of the University of Cambridge.

It furthers the University's mission by disseminating knowledge in the pursuit of education, learning, and research at the highest international levels of excellence.

www.cambridge.org
Information on this title: www.cambridge.org/9781009001205
DOI: 10.1017/9781009000420

© Annapurna H. Poduri, Alfred L. George, Jr., Erin L. Heinzen, Daniel Lowenstein, and Sara James 2021

First published 2021

A catalogue record for this publication is available from the British Library.

ISBN 978-1-009-00120-5 Paperback
ISSN 2633-2086 (online)
ISSN 2633-2078 (print)

Additional resources for this publication at www.cambridge.org/poduri.

How We Got to Where We're Going

Elements in Genetics in Epilepsy

DOI: 10.1017/9781009000420
First published online: August 2021

Annapurna H. Poduri
Boston Children's Hospital, Harvard Medical School

Alfred L. George, Jr.
Northwestern University Feinberg School of Medicine

Erin L. Heinzen
University of North Carolina, Chapel Hill

Daniel Lowenstein
University of California, San Francisco

Sara James
Journalist and author

Author for correspondence: Annapurna H. Poduri,
Annapurna.Poduri@childrens.harvard.edu

Abstract: This Element serves as a welcome to the Cambridge Elements Genetics in Epilepsy series. The series editors look forward to sharing with you the story of epilepsy genetics through a series of Elements. They will bring together many voices, by text as well as video, to illustrate the history of epilepsy genetics, the many ongoing efforts in the field, and how they hope to address the still-unanswered questions that command the attention of all of us and our colleagues across the globe.

Keywords: epilepsy, genetics, epilepsy genetics, neurogenetics, precision medicine

ISBNs: 9781009001205 (PB), 9781009000420 (OC)
ISSNs: 2633-2086 (online), 2633-2078 (print)

Contents

Supplementary video is available at
www.cambridge.org/poduri.

Contributors

Samuel F. Berkovic AM, MD, FAA, FRACP, FRS
*Laureate Professor, Department of Medicine, University of Melbourne;
Director, Epilepsy Research Centre, Austin Health*

1 Welcome and Introduction

Annapurna H. Poduri, MD, MPH
Boston Children's Hospital, Harvard Medical School

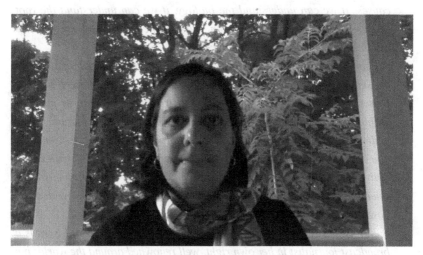

Video 1: Annapurna H. Poduri, MD, MPH. Video available at
www.cambridge.org/poduri.

Video 1 transcript

[Ann Poduri, MD, MPH] Welcome to the Cambridge Elements Genetics in Epilepsy Series. I am Ann Poduri. I am a pediatric neurologist and translational researcher at Boston Children's Hospital, where I direct the Epilepsy Genetics Program. I am joined by Al George, Erin Heinzen, Dan Lowenstein, and Sara James. Together, we are looking forward to sharing with you the story of epilepsy genetics.

One in 26 people will have epilepsy in their lifetime, and for the majority of these individuals who have not had a stroke, or a tumor, or some other acquired cause for the epilepsy – their recurrent, unprovoked seizures – we know today that genetic causes are at play. In some individuals we can identify these causes, and in others we are still searching for them. Together, we'll bring to you the story of how we got here as a field; how genome discovery and careful phenotyping, and bringing together families and individuals with epilepsy, led to those first discoveries of genes responsible for epilepsy. That proof of principle combined with basic science research, animal models, and cellular models have driven the field forward, both to pursue additional genetic causes of epilepsy and also to pursue precise diagnoses for patients that we hope will lead to precise treatments for patients with epilepsy.

For those of us who see patients in clinic, we are all too familiar with the idea that many of our patients continue to have seizures; in fact, one in three patients with epilepsy continue to have seizures despite modern medical treatment. Knowing that, we are even more motivated to find causes. If we can understand the biology, if we can understand the root causes of epilepsy, we can then pursue specific treatments, precise treatments – precision medicine for epilepsy.

Our series will be a series of Elements. Elements are akin to small books or small symposia, where each chapter will be a different talk or presentation. These will be presented in traditional format, in print or online with text and figures, but we are going to add a feature to the series that we think will be special: We'll bring you the experts from their offices and their homes. We'll bring you the voices of families and individuals with epilepsy, to bring you not only the excitement for scientific discovery but also the passion for the field, the why, and the how, and the where are we going.

In this first Element, an introductory overview, Sara will start. Sara is a broadcast journalist in her own right, well renowned around the world; but she is going to bring us first her family's story, the story of her daughter who has a genetic epilepsy that has impacted her life and the life of their whole family. Through the series, Sara will put on her broadcast journalist hat and interview many of our experts, bringing you their voices and their perspectives.

Dan Lowenstein, Professor of Neurology at the University of California, San Francisco, is an expert in the field of genetic epilepsy who has had many leadership roles – as Principal Investigator of the Epilepsy Phenome-Genome Project and Epi4K consortia, President of the Genomics Commission of the ILAE, the International League Against Epilepsy, and current and active member of many, many consortia. Dan brings us not only history himself, but in this first Element he'll bring us Sam Berkovic, another luminary in the field, to tell the story of how we got here, some of the origin stories in our field and in our story of epilepsy genetics.

Al George, at the Northwestern Feinberg School of Medicine, Chair of Pharmacology, will bring to us an additional thread to the story, that of collaboration across institutions. Al will outline for us many of the gene discoveries in epilepsy that have come about through extensive collaboration between clinical researchers and basic researchers, between institutions and across continents. We're looking forward to hearing from Al, not only in this Element but in future Elements about his own and other channel-related work involving epilepsy.

Finally, in this first introductory Element, Erin Heinzen will talk to us about the technologies that have driven gene discovery. Erin is an Associate Professor of Pharmacy and Genetics at the University of North Carolina, Chapel Hill. Her own early work stems from finding copy number variants associated with epilepsy, and more recently she's been driving research in somatic mutations in focal epilepsy, particularly malformations of cortical development. In this introduction, Erin is going to walk us through a history of genomics, how that has applied to epilepsy, and how we've been able to harness genomic discovery to push the envelope in terms of discovering causes for patients today. We know that many patients who have presumed genetic epilepsies still do not have identifiable causes, and Erin will talk to us in this Element and in future Elements as well about how driving technology forward will also help us move our field forward.

We hope we'll be able to bring to you a collection of voices and a collection of stories that together will tell the story of the genetics of epilepsy. Some of our Elements will focus on single genes and will bring to you patients, families, clinical researchers, basic scientists, and clinical trialists to talk about how the stories have emerged and moved forward from the early gene discovery to precision medicine today. Other Elements will talk about genetic epilepsies that are less well formed and that are not yet treated with precise mechanisms, an aspirational view to where we hope to be.

Together, we're extremely excited to be able to do this, to tell this story through multiple Elements, and to invite you to be part of the story. We can't tell you enough how much we appreciate your being interested in the series, and we hope that you'll send us feedback and communicate with us as we move forward, telling the story today and as it unfolds in the future. Welcome again.

On behalf of our Editorial Team, welcome to the Cambridge Elements Genetics in Epilepsy Series. We look forward to sharing with colleagues, students, researchers, clinicians, patients, and families the story of epilepsy genetics through a series of Elements. The Elements will be a series of publications focused on topics in epilepsy genetics, from genetic strategies to basic research to precision medicine. My colleagues and I will bring together many voices, by text as well as video, to illustrate the history of epilepsy genetics, the many ongoing efforts in the field, and how we hope to address the still-unanswered questions that command the attention of all of us and our colleagues across the globe.

What will the Genetics in Epilepsy series cover?

One in twenty-six people have epilepsy, defined as recurrent, unprovoked seizures, and often associated with related conditions that can equally affect quality of life. The field of epilepsy genetics centers around a drive to understand *why* – what lies behind the majority of epilepsy that is not readily explained by stroke, tumor, or other acquired causes? Further, we seek to know how understanding epilepsy's precise genetic causes can move us from a past and present dominated by empiric, trial-and-error treatment without regard to cause toward a future of precision medicine for epilepsy.

We will cover the many steps on the path to precision medicine for epilepsy with a patient-centered approach: enrollment and phenotyping of people with epilepsy, sequencing of DNA using ever-evolving technologies, variant interpretation and reinterpretation, basic laboratory research in neuroscience to understand how seizures arise and propagate in the setting of genetic variants, the development of clinically relevant animal and cellular models, identification of treatment strategies, preclinical trials, and treatment trials. The field relies on patients willing to participate in research, clinician investigators, genomic scientists, and basic and translational neuroscientists. We will see through many examples how teams that come together can drive forward cutting-edge science that is beginning to have an impact on patients with genetic epilepsy.

Our approach to Elements

We are approaching each Element as a mini-symposium, with contributors from multiple disciplines focusing on a common topic within epilepsy genetics. We aim to share the story of epilepsy genetics through a mixture of traditional text, figures, and tables with the addition of videos to bring the experts and their stories directly to the reader. We hope we will be able to introduce our exceptional colleagues and to convey our passion for the field by sharing some of the stories behind the work that make our growing field so rich.

Each Element in the Genetics of Epilepsy series will bring together multiple perspectives through complementary sections, for example, focused on a given gene or pathway:

(1) Patient, Family, and/or Foundation perspective
(2) Clinical Science

(3) Laboratory Science

(4) Translational Research and the Status of Treatment

Once we have addressed the first overview topics and cover several individual genes, we will begin the task of adding new information and reflecting on past hypotheses and projections in new editions of Elements. We have many unanswered questions and many, many patients with suspected but not yet specifically determined genetic epilepsies.

Who are we, and how did we get here?

My own interest in epilepsy genetics stems from my clinical experience as a pediatric epileptologist in training, which led me to pursue a career in translational neurogenetics. Our Epilepsy Genetics Program at Boston Children's Hospital focuses on the discovery of germline and mosaic variants in patients with epilepsy, returning results to patients, and modeling epilepsy genes in zebrafish and cell-based models with a goal of achieving precision medicine for patients with epilepsy.

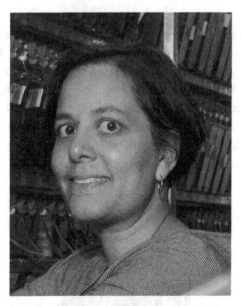

As Lead Editor for the Genetics in Epilepsy series, I have the privilege to work with a highly accomplished team of Deputy Editors, who will lead future Elements focusing on both broad topics in the field and detailed discussions of individual genes, bringing together experts and stakeholders from a variety of disciplines.

- **Daniel Lowenstein, MD** is Professor of Neurology at the University of California, San Francisco. He has served as Principal Investigator of the Epilepsy Phenome/Genome Project and the Epi4K Consortium and is actively engaged in many additional international collaborative initiatives. Dan is past chair and a current member of the Genetics Commission of the International League Against Epilepsy. In this first Element, Dan interviews Dr. Samuel Berkovic of Melbourne, Australia, another luminary in the field of epilepsy genetics whose career has been devoted to advancing our understanding of the genetic causes of epilepsy and translating genetic discovery back to patients.

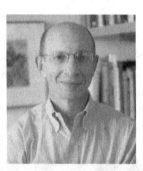

- **Alfred L. George Jr., MD** is Professor and Chair of Pharmacology at the Northwestern University Feinberg School of Medicine. He directs the Channelopathy-associated Epilepsy Research Center without Walls, supported by the National Institutes of Neurological Disorders and Stroke, connecting patient variants with bench science. In this first Element, Al will bring us a state of the field, including the discovery of individual genes and chromosomal loci associated with epilepsy, highlighting the success of large-scale collaborative networks of researchers.

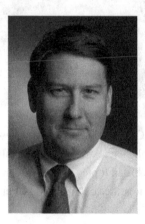

- **Erin L. Heinzen, PharmD, PhD** is Associate Professor of Pharmacy and Genetics at the University of North Carolina at Chapel Hill. She has served as Principal Investigator of the Sequencing, Biostatistics & Bioinformatics Core of the Epi4K Consortium. She is actively engaged in research into somatic mosaic mutation in epilepsy and identifying the mechanisms underlying *SLC35A2* epilepsy. Erin will provide an overview of genomic technologies that have driven forward genetic discovery in epilepsy. Hand in hand with decades of ascertainment and phenotyping of patients with epilepsy, the genomic revolution has led to a revolution in our understanding of the causes of epilepsy.

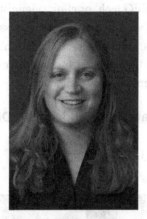

- We are joined by Associate Editor **Sara James** of Melbourne, Australia. Sara is a renowned broadcast journalist who has joined our team to help us tell the evolving story of epilepsy genetics. Sara is also an advocate for research in epilepsy and community–academic partnerships in genetic epilepsy; she is Vice President of the *KCNQ2* Cure Alliance and a co-founder of Genetic Epilepsy Team Australia. We begin this first Element with Sara's personal perspective as a parent of a child with genetic epilepsy as well as her efforts to channel her own professional expertise to rally communities and move toward progress in genetic epilepsies that will translate into improved treatment and quality of life for people with epilepsy.

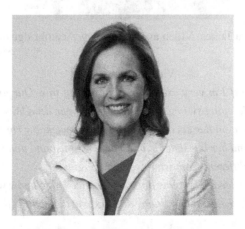

An invitation to join us on our journey in epilepsy genetics

Ours is a story of science, medicine, discovery, and partnerships, and we invite you to "meet" many of our colleagues through this series as they provide detailed reviews of this complex and quickly advancing field. We look forward to the opportunity to present our story in this new format to you. Whether you are a patient with epilepsy, the family member of a patient with epilepsy, a student, trainee, or an experienced researcher, physician, genetic counselor, nurse practitioner, nurse, EEG tech, or clinic administrator, we hope you will find value in the questions we ask and how we address them as a community.

Our whole team shares tremendous excitement about emerging genomic discovery in epilepsy and the potential for this discovery to change the way we approach patients' diagnoses and treatments.

2 Of Pirate Ships and Sailing Dreams

Sara James
Journalist and author

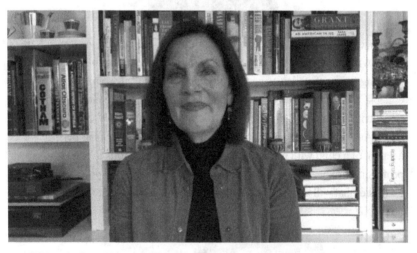

Video 2: Sara James. Video available at www.cambridge.org/poduri.

Video 2 transcript

[Sara James] I'm very excited to be a part of this. Our family's journey with genetic epilepsy began when our younger daughter was born. She had a seizure on her second day of life, and we knew right then that her journey – and her big sister's and that of my husband and me – was going to be very different from what we had imagined.

We really needed to know answers. We needed to know what was going wrong, and we talked to so many doctors; but at the time, there really were no answers. It would be seven years, by which point we were living here in Australia, before we got a diagnosis. It came from Professor Ingrid Scheffer, and she told us that our daughter Jacqui has something called KCNQ2 encephalopathy.

Well, when we heard that, it just sounded like a bunch of numbers and letters. I'm a journalist by training, so I decided to try to reach out to other parents; and I quickly discovered that other families had exactly the same idea. We connected and created something called KCNQ2 Cure, and that connection was powerful. We learned that there was a lot that we shared.

The same thing happened yet again here in Australia, when my husband and I joined with a couple of other families and created something called GETA, Genetic Epilepsy Team Australia, because we've decided that collaborating is really the way forward, and there is so much more that unites our various different genetic epilepsies than there is that's different between them.

I think the final lesson that I've learned is that we have to communicate. We need to share what it is that we've learned, whether it's the latest piece of research or maybe a behavior strategy that will help; because it's a challenging journey, isn't it? Our daughter has a seizure disorder, she has an intellectual disorder, and she has autism; and while it might be different between all the different genetic epilepsies, they all come with a grab bag of challenges. So that connection, that collaboration, and that communication are crucial, no matter where you live around the world. Because genetic epilepsy doesn't recognize any borders.

That's why I'm excited to be a part of this. It's the next step in my journey, and I'm thrilled to participate – as a journalist, as an advocate, and as a mom.

Jacqui, decked out in scarlet scarf, belted white blouse, and eye patch, sits astride a chestnut mare. A black hat decorated with a skull and crossbones is perched on her head. She carries a cardboard ship, complete with waves, like a gigantic handbag.

"Say cheese!" someone shouts. Jacqui brandishes her toy sword with a grin that makes her eyebrow-penciled moustache wiggle.

Our daughter is dressed to compete in a gymkhana, a kid-friendly equestrian show held by the local pony club near our home in the Macedon Ranges of Australia. She makes a splendid girl pirate, I decide – a modern-day Jacquotte Delahaye, the notorious seventeenth-century buccaneer known as "Back from the Dead Red." Or maybe I'm just another stage mom. I want my pirate to win.

That's when I realize Jacqui already has won. She's happy, she's healthy, and she's here.

Jacqui was born on August 28, 2004, after a fraught pregnancy and arduous delivery. Our tiny girl looked beautiful, but it alarmed me that she didn't cry. Her big sister Sophie had announced her arrival with a lusty yodel, then took stock of her surroundings with a beady-eyed stare.

I said a little prayer that Jacqui would be all right.

But it wasn't that simple.

Jacqui had her first seizure on her second day of life. Then she had another. And another. It is nearly impossible to express the horror of witnessing a tiny baby convulse, turning breathless and blue. Especially when that baby is your own.

Jacqui received excellent care in the NICU of a top-notch New York City hospital. That included a battery of tests, none of which explained what was wrong. Men and women in white coats fluttered about her. I found their scientific pronouncements impenetrable as the chatter of gulls.

But not for long. Like so many parents of children born with a rare disease, I soon harnessed my professional skills to help our daughter. I was a correspondent at NBC News. My husband Andrew also worked in media. We would be reporters. We would reach out to expert doctors, scientists, and therapists as well as other parents like us.

Jacqui spent more than a month in the hospital. But it would take seven years before we received a diagnosis. By then, we'd moved to my husband's home turf and lived in the countryside near Melbourne in Australia. I tracked down a world-renowned expert in genetic epilepsy. Thanks to the brilliant Professor Ingrid Scheffer of the University of Melbourne, Jacqui was one of the first people in the world diagnosed with KCNQ2.

KCNQ2 Developmental and Epileptic Encephalopathy (KCNQ2 DEE) is a mouthful of a diagnosis. This genetic epilepsy is linked to a tiny but profound fault in the potassium channel. KCNQ2 DEE causes epilepsy, an intellectual disability, and in some cases – like Jacqui's – autism.

Jacqui's pirate costume suits her. She's funny and feisty and fearless. But no one would call her an easy child. There are times when I've felt metaphorically ordered to walk the plank – dunked in deep water and gasping. Our daughter's behavioral challenges require constant one-on-one management. They have landed her in the hospital.

Genetic epilepsy is tough. For children. For their brothers and sisters. For their parents, and for their grandparents, too.

We count ourselves lucky that Jacqui's epilepsy is well controlled. Many people with genetic epilepsy have frequent, devastating seizures. It's a battle to walk, to talk, to learn, to live. Many in our community are nonverbal and require mobility assistance. Every year, children die from this dreadful disease.

I marvel to see my girl on that horse. At four, she didn't have enough core strength to slide down a slide. Now, after many years participating with Riding for Disabled Australia, she can take a trail ride. And while Jacqui still finds it hard to answer a question, she always tells us what she thinks. If a cell phone rings, she's liable to sing out, "Siri! Put a sock in it!" Making people laugh is her greatest joy.

My girl pirate didn't ask to sail on this ship and neither did we. Nobody does. But there are choices.

We've discovered that the best way to navigate uncharted waters is to sail with a first-rate crew. This isn't as difficult as it sounds. There's a magnetism that attracts parents of children born with rare diseases and disorders. There is so much that doesn't need to be said. Our talents can complement one another, as I discovered when I signed on with Jim Johnson, Scotty Sims, and Caroline Loewy to found KCNQ2 Cure Alliance more than five years ago. We host an annual family and professional summit. These are big, noisy affairs that feel like a family reunion. We laugh a lot. We have an active Facebook page and support, even drive, scientific research.

We know that science matters – for our kids, and those yet to be born. My husband Andrew and I created the annual KCNQ2 Cure New Horizons in Science Dinner in Melbourne to celebrate world-leading scientists and raise money for a cure. Andrew and I also joined with Australian husband-and-wife teams Kris Pierce and David Cunnington, and Danielle and Danny Williams to form GETA – Genetic Epilepsy Team Australia. Our children have different genetic epilepsies, but there is much we share. We are convinced we can get farther by uniting families living with rare genetic epilepsies to form a larger group that has more weight with researchers and governments.

Over the past 15 years, there have been stormy passages and moments of heart-wrenching beauty. Fellow parents, therapists, doctors, and scientists are now dear friends. I long ago gave up my wish for smooth sailing, though I smile with relief when it sometimes occurs. And I take heart from my fearless pirate and my mates. The treasure we seek is a cure. But until we find it, we're in this. Together.

Links

KCNQ2 CURE
www.kcnq2cure.org
Genetic Epilepsy Team Australia (GETA)
www.geneticepilepsyteam.com.au/

Sara James' website
www.sarajames.com.au
A Place for Us/AUSTRALIAN STORY/ABC Australia
https://www.youtube.com/watch?v=5Krl6H8fw4M#action=share

3 Epilepsy Genetics – A Brief History

Daniel Lowenstein, MD
University of California, San Francisco

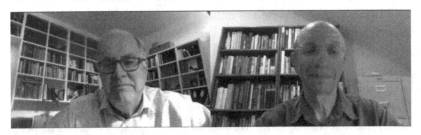

Video 3: Samuel Berkovic, MD and Daniel Lowenstein, MD.
Video available at www.cambridge.org/poduri.

Video 3 transcript

[Dan Lowenstein, MD (DL)] Welcome, everyone, to this part of the first edition of the Cambridge Elements series on the Genetics of Epilepsy. My name is Dan Lowenstein, and I'm a Professor of Neurology at the University of California San Francisco. I am delighted to host an interview with a colleague and friend, Dr. Sam Berkovic. Dr. Berkovic is the Laureate Professor in the Department of Medicine in the University of Melbourne, and he's the Director of the Epilepsy Research Center at Austin Health. He received his medical training at the University of Melbourne and spent three years at the Montreal Neurologic Institute. He's a clinician-researcher with a special interest in establishing close research links with basic scientists; and his group, together with molecular genetic collaborators in Adelaide and Germany, discovered the first gene for epilepsy in 1995, and subsequently have been involved in the discovery of many of the known epilepsy genes. He heads a large Australian research program grant, integrating genetic, imaging, and physiological studies in epilepsy, and he was elected a Fellow of the Royal Society in 2007 and an international member of the National Academy of Medicine in 2017. Together with Ingrid Scheffer, he was awarded the Prime Minister's Prize for Science in 2014. In the interest of full disclosure, I should let you, the viewers, know that Dr. Berkovic and

I are very close professional friends. For that reason, we're going to be a bit informal; I'm going to refer to him as my friend Sam. So, Sam, welcome; thank you so much for participating in this inaugural edition of the Genetics series for Cambridge.

[Sam Berkovic, MD (SB)] *Thank you, Dan, it's a pleasure to talk to you.*

[DL] *The goal here is to give the viewers a sense of the development of the field, because you've been so much a centerpiece of the work that's gone on throughout your entire career. So let's dive in. For starters, what initially drew you into a career as a physician-scientist interested in the genetics of epilepsy?*

[SB] *I think mentorship's got a lot to do with it. I trained in medicine. I was drawn to neurology largely because there was a charismatic leader of neurology in my hospital, Peter Bladin, and he got me interested. I did an internship with him, and I saw he was working in epilepsy, which certainly in Australia and in many other parts of the world was very much a Cinderella specialty; nobody was particularly interested in it except for very few people, and he was the leader of epilepsy in Australia and saw a future there. I didn't work on genetics or have any training in genetics, but he sent me to Montreal at the MNI where I had a wonderful three years with Fred and Eva Andermann; they were a team of epileptologists and geneticists, and that really interested me. I saw that as a way that myself as a clinician – and I prided myself on my clinical training – could understand something about basic biology just by observing clinical patterns. That's how I got fascinated by genetics.*

[DL] *Did the Andermanns encourage you specifically into this area of epilepsy?*

[SB] *They worked in Quebec, where there's a lot of consanguinity, and they were interested, in addition to epilepsy, in many of the other classic heritable diseases that have seizures as part of them, and I went on field trips with them and saw families and sort of learnt how to do it by observing them. I also had privileged access to a famous series of twins collected by William Lennox in Boston. Eva Andermann happened to have the files of Lennox, the monozygotic twin files, and she suggested I look through them and see what I could glean from them. I just found this a fantastic clinical insight – when you've got no idea about the causation of something, and you see it pop up in monozygotic twins, it sort of screams at you that this is genetic. I thought this was a very cool way of understanding biology as a clinician, and that drew me to it. When I came back to Australia, which had no track record in epilepsy genetics, it seemed to me that a twin study was a good way to go, and that's how*

I started. Then we moved into looking at families, and I was probably lucky because the structure in Australia – of most of the population living in a few big cities – meant that the families weren't as distributed as they might have been in some other places, and particularly in North America or even Europe. We were able to gather together large families with epilepsy and try to work it out, and that led to some of our early discoveries.

[DL] So, we're going back 30–40 years. What was it like when you discovered the first true epilepsy gene? I guess it was in the years leading up to 1995, right?

[SB] Yes, I think it was – I forget the exact date, but it was sort of toward the end of '94, and Ingrid Scheffer and I had collected this very large family with nocturnal frontal lobe epilepsy. The science of that as clinicians was getting an absolutely large pedigree, because that was the clue to enable the genetic technique at the time – which was linkage analysis, putting together a jigsaw puzzle of the family and figuring out which marker is segregated with the disease – to work. This was Ingrid's PhD, which I supervised, and we got together this very large family. Then our colleagues in Adelaide, particularly Grant Sutherland and John Mulley, figured out where the linkage was. At that time, relatively few genes were known in terms of their location, but we were lucky that where this gene mapped to on the long arm of chromosome 20, there was an interesting candidate, the nicotinic receptor, and that turned out to be the gene. That gene was being studied by Ortrud Steinlein in Germany. We contacted her, and that was kind of the magic of one of those scientific collaborations. I remember, I was sitting in my study at home when she rang me and said, I think I found a change in this gene, and what it was. I had some papers on my desk about the gene and I quickly looked up the amino acid chains that she was describing, and that was sort of a magical moment for me as a clinical scientist, because it all made sense, and that was great. We had a number of other similar discoveries in other ion channels, as did other groups around the world, and that's how things got rolling with the initial discoveries of epilepsy's channelopathies, at least in some of these large families.

[DL] Were the subsequent discoveries just as exciting as the first? I kind of assume there's nothing like the first.

[SB] Oh, yes; your first child's always got something special, but you love them all. I mean, in the big picture, nicotinic receptors – we thought maybe this is the answer to everything, but as it's turned out it's a real rarity, and I think that's still true although it's important. Some of the *other subsequent channel discoveries have been, I think, more important in terms of numbers, but the concept was a very important one to have got the first building blocks for.*

[DL] Now, before asking you a little bit about the current setting of epilepsy genetics and looking forward, let's go back a bit. I know you've had an interest in Lennox both in terms of the studies that you referred to already as well as him as a person, and that brings us into the earlier part of the twentieth century. Tell us a little bit about what was going on in epilepsy genetics around that time in terms of progress or challenges to progress.

[SB] Yes, the history of epilepsy genetics is interesting and complicated. Hippocrates recognized that epilepsy had a genetic component, and then when neurology developed to some extent in the nineteenth century in the UK and in Europe, the writers at that time generally recognized that epilepsy had a big genetic component and that family history was important. But in the early part of the twentieth century, it kind of wasn't important, and this really puzzled me. Lennox was, I think, the person who studied this most thoroughly, first of all by twins and also by family studies that he had very large numbers, and his writing showed that there was this major component. Yet he specifically said that there is a genetic component to epilepsy, but it's not as important as in other diseases, it's not the big issue. Retrospectively, I'd never understood this, but the way I've analyzed this, there were two reasons for this. One is a genuine biological reason, in that the Mendelian types of disorders, the Mendelian epilepsies are actually relatively rare. What we learned in high school about Mendel and his peas, and about classical metabolic disorders that are inherited or other disorders – that, for the most part, doesn't apply to epilepsy, except to some of the exceptions we and others worked on early with these large families. For the most part, epilepsy genetics is complex. In other words, the risk to first-degree relatives is lower than in classical disorders. But having said that, that's true of most diseases. The man in the street knows that heart disease runs in families, might run in his family, as does asthma and diabetes, and epilepsy also runs in families but it wasn't talked about. I think the reason for that is the terrible stain that eugenics had on medicine and society in general, that people with epilepsy were positively discriminated against, they were murdered by the Nazis. Eugenics, which started off as an apparently benign and beneficial thing to society, of course wasn't, and the things that the people who wrote and thought then would certainly not be accepted now in our current ethical framework. But I think eugenics

and the terrible things that happened in the midpart of the century made it very difficult to talk about a family history of epilepsy. They didn't want to talk about it, the lay societies didn't want to talk about it because it was such an awful stain. But science has the truth, and it took the march of that to enable groups to apply for grants, get grants, and study this in a systematic way and talk about the fact that genetics was important. In fact, it turned out to be more important than we realized, now with the discovery of de novo mutations, which do not show themselves in families or even indeed often in twins.

[DL] Right, of course. We both know the stigma related to epilepsy persists around the world, but thank goodness we have found ourselves beyond the era of the type of stigma that was associated with the period in the twentieth century.

[SB] Yes.

[DL] The goal of the Cambridge Elements series is to try to identify for readers the state of the art, of the field, and that's what viewers can expect in the coming years. So, Sam, what do you see as the main opportunities and barriers to progress in epilepsy genetics going forward here in 2020?

[SB] The first thing to say is I think there's been enormous progress by multiple groups around the world and particularly some of the large collaborative groups, which have been essential in cracking open some of these puzzles; but puzzles still remain. As I've already mentioned, I think one of the big discoveries has been this importance of de novo mutations, particularly in the epileptic encephalopathies, these children who grow up to adults if they don't die of SUDEP [sudden unexplained death in epilepsy] or the illness, one of the major burdens of epilepsy in all our clinics and obviously enormous burdens to their families. Understanding this has been, I think, a major breakthrough. That continues on, almost monthly or weekly, that new genes are found and subtleties to improving treatment discovered. The big unsolved question in my mind is genetic contribution to the commoner epilepsies, particularly the generalized epilepsies but also some of the focal epilepsies; and how much of this is polygenic and how much of this is due to rare variants we're still trying to sort out. But I think the current big studies going on will or have already shed some light and will clarify it even more in the next few years. The big challenge is transitioning this to precision medicine and benefits to the patients. That's already happening in terms of diagnosis and in certain cases where very specific treatments are shown by the genetics, but the big impact we hope is yet to come and hopefully not too far away. I'm very excited about some of the new

potential molecular therapies such as antisense oligonucleotides, which have been shown to work in things like spinal muscular atrophy, and there's now good evidence in animal models that they work in some of the human epilepsies engineered in mice, and hopefully we'll see trials of that in humans. That will be truly spectacular, to have gone from not understanding the disease was genetic at all to finding the gene and then developing a specific therapeutic. So I see that as sort of incredibly exciting and interesting, and that's, of course, not the only precision medicine approach. But if you would have asked me five years ago did I think there was likelihood to be a treatment that would be given with Dravet syndrome or SCN2A or something, I would have thought it would be a little bit further off, but it seems to be very close, and I think that's very exciting.

[DL] I'm going to ask you one last question, and that is sort of bringing it back to you and your own personal odyssey in all this. You've had a truly extraordinary impact on the field. It strikes me as something that's been a very fulfilling and enriching life for you, and so many of us admire what you've done. In looking back at everything – the caring for patients, the training, the training of others – what would you say has been the most gratifying part of the work that you've done in this field?

[SB] I think as a clinician it's when you bring it back to the patient. I find intellectually the most rewarding thing is if I see a patient in the clinic and I'm doing my best to make the diagnosis and give the best treatment; but if I can then ask myself the question, what is this patient telling me about the biology, and can I figure something out and give something back? If you can complete that cycle, which may take many years, to me that's the most rewarding thing; that's sort of solving a clinical research puzzle, which you can't do in a single consultation or even over a little while, but is a process over years. That probably gives me the most satisfaction. In the clinical research sphere, that happens – you recruit a patient or a family and you work on it and you work on it and you work on it, and then you're able to bring it back to the family; and they're usually very, very grateful. I find that very, very gratifying.

[DL] The number of patients and families who have benefited from the work that you and your colleagues have done over the years, plus the number of patients who are going to benefit from the groundwork and the advances that you and others have made, is truly incalculable, and I can just imagine the gratitude they feel. With that, I'm going to thank you, Sam, for spending time with me and with our viewers for just a delightful interview. It is a pleasure to have this opportunity, and thank you.

[SB] Thank you so much, Dan.

The notion that epilepsy has a genetic basis goes back to at least the time of Hippocrates in roughly 400 BC, when the first known monograph on epilepsy, entitled "On the Sacred Disease," included heredity as a cause.[1] This concept was also advanced in Arabic and Latin writings in the Middle Ages, where a proposed explanation for the observation of "inheritance" was the transfer of any disease of the father "through his seed." Throughout this early history, the relative contribution of heredity across all forms of epilepsy was varied and unclear. Some authors (including Hippocrates) implied it was a common cause, as was the case with many other diseases. John Russell Reynolds, in his textbook on epilepsy published in 1861, wrote that the "current belief among ancient writers, and among many at present day, is that epilepsy is pre-eminently an [sic] hereditary affliction."[2] On the other hand, Leuret's 1843 description of the causes of epilepsy ascribed heredity in only one of 66 patients, while more than half of the cases were explained by "fear . . . masturbation . . . or drunkenness."[3]

The first formal scientific demonstration of the influence of genetics in epilepsy came from William Lennox, who published a series of papers in the mid-twentieth century on epilepsy in twins and families.[4] By looking at the differences between monozygotic and dizygotic twins, and differentiating those with and without brain lesions, he showed that, for twins without brain lesions, there was 85 percent concordance for monozygotic twins and 16 percent concordance for dizygotic twins. For those with brain lesions, concordance dropped to 27 percent for mono-zygotic twins, suggesting that genes play a prominent role in the non-acquired epilepsies. These observations were followed by a growing number of population-based, epidemiological studies, which clearly established the role of inheritance in epilepsy. For example, in a study based in Rochester, MN, of all women with epilepsy who bore children between 1922 and 1976, Annegers et al. found that for individuals with siblings with epilepsy, the incidence of epilepsy was 3.2 times higher than expected in the normal population.[5] In a subsequent population-based study of 1,092 relatives of patients with childhood-onset epilepsy, the relative risk of epilepsy was 2.5 in their siblings and 6.7 in their children.[6]

Supported by this knowledge of a major role of genetics as a determinant of epilepsy, the next phase of discovery, which continues to this day, falls into the domain of the "gene hunters." An initial method for homing in on genes was through linkage analysis, which looks at the inheritance of phenotypic traits in families by taking advantage of the co-segregation of nearby regions of DNA sequences during meiosis. Using this method, Leppert et al. were the first to identify in 1989 a gene region associated with a pure form of epilepsy with an autosomal dominant inheritance pattern, finding linkage of benign familial neo-natal convulsions to chromosome 20.[7] (It took another nine years to determine that the mutation was in a gene encoding a potassium channel.[8]) But the honor of being the first to discover a specific "epilepsy" gene goes to Steinlein and colleagues in 1995,[9] who collected detailed phenotypic information on a very large Australian family with autosomal dominant frontal lobe epilepsy, and, based on initial localization of the gene on chromosome 20 through linkage analysis, were able to identify the specific causative mutation in the neuronal nicotinic acetylcholine receptor α4 subunit.

Subsequent studies of other forms of epilepsy in families, such as generalized epilepsy with febrile seizures plus (GEFS+) and autosomal dominant nocturnal frontal lobe epilepsy (also termed sleep-related hypermotor epilepsy), led to the discovery of mutations in a variety of genes encoding ion channels and to the intuitively appealing idea that most forms of genetic epilepsy were in a category of diseases known as "channelopathies." However, although it is true that genes encoding ion channels constitute a major class of epilepsy genes, we now know that there are numerous other genes causing epilepsy, including those encoding synaptic machinery, transcription factors, and neuronal development. Another important insight that emerged during this time was that the assignment of a specific gene to a specific epilepsy syndrome was not going to be as straightforward as in many other genetic disorders. It quickly became evident that mutations in different genes could cause similar epilepsy syndromes (locus heterogeneity), and the same mutation in a given gene could yield various phenotypes (variable expressivity).

At the start of the twenty-first century, the expectation was that further genetic studies of larger populations of people with more-common forms of epilepsy (e.g., not necessarily familial) would see an ongoing rise in the number of identified epilepsy genes. This was the beginning of the era of genome-wide association studies (GWAS), in which there is a search for small genomic variations, called single nucleotide polymorphisms or SNPs, that occur more frequently in people with a particular disease than in people without the disease. This method had proven itself in other diseases such as Parkinson's disease and diabetes; but, at least initially, this was not the case with epilepsy, in large part due to the lack of sufficiently large cohorts needed to achieve statistical significance of a causal association. Fortunately, however, this so-called "dark age" of epilepsy genetics was relatively short-lived, ending in 2012 with the first successful association study of Idiopathic Generalized Epilepsy (IGE) by the European EPICURE Consortium, which showed a significant association with known epilepsy genes such as *SCN1A* and *CHRM3*, along with a number of other non-channel genes.[10] Another useful consequence of the GWAS effort was the ability to detect copy number variants (CNVs), which are small regions of either missing or additional stretches of DNA. CNVs, such as microdeletions in the chromosome 15 region 15q13.3, have been causally linked to certain forms of epilepsy, and numerous studies have shown that people with more-severe forms of epilepsy have an overall greater number of CNVs than controls, similar to what has been observed in studies of people with autism and intellectual disability.

The past decade has seen a major inflection point in epilepsy genetics as a result of rapidly evolving technological advances in DNA sequencing (next-generation sequencing, or NGS), which have enabled gene hunters to study virtually the entire coding sequence of DNA (whole exome sequencing) or the entire genome (whole genome sequencing). A key observation that emerged from the analysis of larger and larger numbers of sequences was the unexpected amount of genetic variation in the human genome, which increased the likelihood that the more-common forms of non-acquired epilepsy are explained by more-complex genetic patterns, for example, a consequence of polygenic effects. Also surprising was the number of so-called de novo mutations in the genome (i.e., variants not inherited from either parent but instead arising from new mutations in the ovum of the mother or the sperm of the father). This finding, paired with the observation that most forms of severe early onset epilepsy, so called "epileptic encephalopathies," are not inherited, led to a series of important discoveries showing that a substantial number of non-acquired epileptic encephalopathies are, indeed, due to de novo mutations or copy number variants in genes encoding ion channels, synaptic proteins, and numerous others. In fact, it is currently estimated that well more than 50 percent of all non-acquired epileptic encephalopathies are due to de novo mutations, a remarkable advance given that a very small fraction could be explained a decade earlier. Important progress has also been made as a result of discoveries that somatic mosaic variants (i.e., genetic variants present in some cells in a given tissue but not others, resulting from mutations that arose after the one-cell stage during development) cause certain forms of focal epilepsy with and without abnormalities identifiable by neuroimaging.

The other area of recent, exciting progress has been in the application of next-generation sequencing to the study of the more-common forms of epilepsy such as genetic generalized epilepsy (GGE) and non-acquired localization-related epilepsy. The earlier GWAS efforts made it abundantly clear such research would require amassing very large cohorts of well-phenotyped patients. This understanding prompted epilepsy clinicians and scientists around the globe to organize into multidisciplinary, collaborative teams, and many important advances have come from groups such as the International League Against Epilepsy Consortium on Complex Genetics, EuroEpinomics, the Epilepsy Phenome/Genome Project, Epi4K, EpiPGX, and, most recently, Epi25, a truly global effort bringing together scores of cohorts from around the world with the goal of analyzing at least 25,000 sequences and associated phenotypes. Interestingly, initial results from the study of these large cohorts is revealing that the same genes, and even the same variants, are involved in both rare and common forms of epilepsy, suggesting they are not distinct entities as was originally thought.

Thus, the history of epilepsy genetics follows a pattern similar to that of many other domains in medicine. The role of heredity has been recognized since antiquity, the patterns of inheritance were refined throughout the twentieth century, and gene discovery quickly emerged once the tools for gene sequencing became available. We now find ourselves in the era of complex genetics, and current and future work will require the study of even larger populations of well-phenotyped subjects, more-refined tools for precise sequencing and interpretation of the whole genome, and exploration of the intricate mechanisms involved in the expression of genes and related downstream events that ultimately control protein function.

4 Exploiting Collaborative Networks in Epilepsy Research

Alfred L. George, Jr., MD
Northwestern University Feinberg School of Medicine

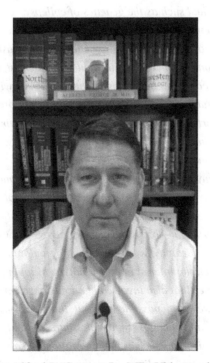

Video 4: Alfred L. George, Jr., MD. Video available at
www.cambridge.org/poduri.

Video 4 transcript

[Al George, MD] Hello, I'm Al George, one of the Deputy Editors of the Cambridge Elements series on the Genetics of Epilepsy. I'm also a Professor and Chairman of the Department of Pharmacology at the Northwestern University Feinberg School of Medicine in Chicago. I am delighted to be working with my colleagues Ann Poduri, Dan Lowenstein, and Erin Heinzen, as well as Sara James, on this important initiative.

I've been involved in research in the molecular genetics of human ion channels for more than 30 years. For the past 20 years, we've devoted our laboratory's effort to evaluating the functional consequences of genetic mutations in voltage-gated ion channels in the brain, that are the cause of a variety of monogenic epilepsy syndromes.

Recently we started a Center Without Walls for research in epilepsy, funded by the National Institute of Neurological Disorders and Stroke, and this Center involves 20 investigators and 10 institutions, including 2 companies, across the United States. This Center is a good example of the importance and value of collaborative networks for making important advances in a field such as the genetics of epilepsy.

Indeed, the emergence of collaborative networks, and their importance for making discoveries in epilepsy genetics over the past 20 or more years, is the focus of one chapter in this introductory Element, where we trace the importance of consortia beginning in the mid-1990s with the discovery of the genes for tuberous sclerosis, all the way to the present time with the Herculean efforts of the Epi25 collaborative and their ambitious goal of sequencing exomes from 25,000 persons with epilepsy.

The importance of collaboration in the field of epilepsy cannot be overstated. Many of the genes responsible for monogenic forms of epilepsy, and indeed discoveries related to more genetically complex forms of common epilepsy, have been made possible by this selfless collaboration of hundreds of scientists working in dozens of countries across the world.

This work, importantly, was built upon a foundation laid by the Human Genome Project, the International Haplotype Mapping Project, and other similar initiatives that also involved hundreds of scientists. This work also would not have been possible without the generous funding by both governmental and nongovernmental sources, and the guidance by advocacy organizations such as the International League Against Epilepsy.

I hope you enjoy reading about this evolution of what has become a revolution in the epilepsy genetic field, and will come back to take advantage of this series, where we hope to dive deeper into some of the

very specific genes that have been discovered in the past several years. We
look forward to seeing you in the future, and I hope you enjoy reading about
these discoveries. Thank you.

Scientific advances occur because of many factors. More often than not, multidisciplinary research requires expertise not available in single laboratories or groups. In modern human genetics research, the need to bridge scientific disciplines has driven nontraditional partnerships, as demonstrated by the Human Genome Project,[11] the international haplotype mapping (HapMap) project,[12] and the 1000 Genomes Project,[13] uniting teams of molecular biologists, computer scientists, and experts in laboratory automation that were further catalyzed by academic–industry partnerships. Furthermore, in today's scientific environment, research that sprouts from individual ideas and discoveries is often enabled or accelerated by large-scale projects that provide critical databases, shared resources, and expansive knowledge that can only be acquired through collaborative networks.

The major advances in epilepsy genetics during the past decades can be attributed in part to the emergence of several multinational consortia (Table 1). One of the first demonstrated successes of this approach traces to the discoveries of two major genes for tuberous sclerosis complex, which were first mapped to chromosomes 9 and 16,[14,15] and later identified through positional cloning efforts by the European Chromosome 16 Tuberous Sclerosis Consortium (TSC2), [16] and the TSC1 Consortium (TSC1).[17] Further large-scale efforts devoted to phenotyping, gene mapping, and gene sequencing were later funded by governmental sources such as the National Institutes of Health in the United States, the European Commission, and nongovernmental entities including the European Science Foundation and the Wellcome Trust, along with many other regional philanthropic foundations and agencies. A key driver behind these efforts was the International League Against Epilepsy (ILAE) Commission on Genetics of Epilepsy and the ILAE Consortium on Complex Epilepsies, which helped coordinate efforts to investigate the basis of epilepsies that required large multinational cohorts. Parallel efforts funded by the European Commission provided incentive for groups to work across borders on that continent, which led to the first successful population-based gene mapping studies. This early European effort was led by Thomas Sander at the University of Cologne, who established the EPICURE Consortium.

Table 1 Collaborative networks in epilepsy genetics

Consortium	Web Site or Citation Link
European Chromosome 16 Tuberous Sclerosis Consortium	https://doi.org/10.1016/0092-8674(93)90618-Z
TSC1 Consortium	http://doi.org/10.1126/science.277.5327.805
EPICURE consortium	https://doi.org/10.1111/j.1528-1167.2011.03379.x
EpiGEN	https://doi.org/10.1093/brain/awq130
ILAE Consortium on Complex Epilepsies	www.ilae.org/guidelines/complex-epilepsies
EuroEpinomics-Res	http://archives.esf.org/coordinating-research/eurocores/programmes/euroepinomics.html
EuroEpinomics-CoGIE	http://archives.esf.org/coordinating-research/eurocores/programmes/euroepinomics.html
EpiPGX Consortium	www.epipgx.eu/
Epilepsy Phenome/Genome Project	https://epgp.org/
Epi4K Center without Walls	https://doi.org/10.1111/j.1528-1167.2012.03511.x
Epilepsy and Migraine Integrated Network (EMINet Consortium)	www.ngfn.de/en/epilepsie_und_migr__ne__.html
Epi25 Collaborative	http://epi-25.org/
Center for SUDEP Research	https://sudep.org/sudep-center-without-walls
Epilepsy Bioinformatics Study for Antiepileptogenic Therapy	https://epibios.loni.usc.edu/
Rational Intervention for KCNQ2/3 Epileptic Encephalopathy (RIKEE)	www.rikee.org/
Channelopathy-associated Epilepsy Research Center without Walls	https://epilepsy-channelopathy.org/
Epilepsy Gene Curation Expert Panel (ClinGen)	https://clinicalgenome.org/affiliation/40005/

The EPICURE Consortium conducted two large-scale investigations of GGE including a genome-wide linkage analysis of 379 multiplex families and a GWAS of 3,020 cases and 3,954 controls. The families used in the linkage study had been ascertained by the European partners in the consortium beginning in 1995 and represented the largest familial epilepsy cohort studied at the time. Findings from the first study supported an oligogenic predisposition to GGE with risk alleles mapped to chromosome 5q34, 2q34, and 13q31.3.[18] The GWAS identified two genomic regions (2p16.1, 17q21.32) significantly associated with GGE, as well as independent loci associated with genetic absence epilepsy (2q22.3) and juvenile myoclonic epilepsy (1q43). [10] A suggestive locus near the *SCN1A* gene (q24.3) was also found. This work by the EPICURE Consortium offered the first demonstration of a successful GWAS in epilepsy made possible by this multinational collaboration.

The ILAE Consortium on Complex Epilepsies was born in December 2009 during a meeting of the ILAE Genetics Commission with the goal of enabling successful GWAS through the aggregation of independent cohorts for meta-analysis. This initiative led to successful completion of a GWAS published in 2014 involving 8,696 cases with epilepsy and 26,157 ethnically matched controls from 12 cohorts.[19] The study identified genomic loci near *SCN1A* (2q24.3) and *PCDH7* (4p15.1) as significant among all cases, and an additional signal at 2p16.1 among a subpopulation with GGE. This important work demonstrated that genetic susceptibility for common epilepsies could be identified through an analysis of common genomic variation. An expanded GWAS by the ILAE Consortium involving 15,212 individuals with epilepsy and nearly 30,000 controls revealed 16 mostly novel loci with genome-wide significance.[20] A group of 21 genes with greatest likelihood to account for the associations were enriched in monogenic epilepsy genes and known antiepileptic drug targets. Most of the loci showed association in persons with GGE with common variants explaining a third of the disease susceptibility. A graphical summary of mapped loci is provided in Figure 1.

Concurrent with progress in GWAS of epilepsy, other efforts focused on identifying rare genetic causes of epilepsy were emerging. In Europe, the EuroEPINOMICS initiative was launched with the stated objectives to identify novel epilepsy genes and genetic variants predisposing to epilepsy and drug response, and to unravel molecular pathways. The program began in 2011 with funding commitments from 15 European nations coordinated by the European Science Foundation. Four separate research projects were commissioned, including the Genetics of Rare Epilepsy Syndromes (RES), Genetic Targets of Epileptogenesis and Pharmacoresistance in Brain Glial Cells (Epiglia),

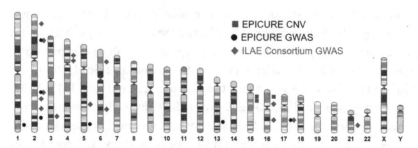

Figure 1 Genomic loci associated with epilepsy. Human chromosome idiograms are decorated with the approximate locations of genomic loci mapped by the EPICURE Consortium or the ILAE Consortium on Complex Epilepsies. The ideogram renderings were obtained from Ryan Collins (https://github.com/RCollins13/HumanIdiogramLibrary) under a Creative Commons license.

Epigenetic Pathomechanisms Promoting Epileptogenesis in Focal and Generalised Epilepsies (EpiGENet), and Complex Genetics of Idiopathic Epilepsies (CoGIE). EuroEPINOMICS-RES, led by Peter De Jonghe from the University of Antwerp, was particularly fruitful with the discovery of several novel epilepsy genes,[21–26] and success in unraveling the phenotypic spectrum of various rare genetic epilepsies.[27–32] CoGIE, led by Holger Lerche at the University of Tübingen, had success later in using exome sequencing to find susceptibility alleles in GGE.

The Epilepsy Phenome/Genome Project (EPGP) ascertained >5,000 extensively phenotyped cases to better understand the genetic basis and clinical features of epilepsy.[33,34] This cohort provided the foundation for the first large-scale exome sequencing project in epilepsy, Epi4K.[35] This sequencing project was launched in 2011 with a new funding mechanism (Centers without Walls for Collaborative Research in the Epilepsies) initiated by NINDS. Epi4K was designed to accelerate progress in unraveling genetic mechanisms underlying common and rare forms of epilepsy by generating exome sequence data for at least 4,000 persons with epilepsy.

An initial focus of Epi4K was a cohort with epileptic encephalopathy including 149 probands with infantile spasms and another 115 with Lennox–Gastaut syndrome and their parents.[36] Analysis of exome sequences identified 329 de novo mutations in several genes that were significantly enriched in these populations. Five genes were previously known to be associated with epileptic encephalopathy (*CDKL5*, *SCN1A*, *SCN2A*, *SCN8A*, *STXBP1*), and four other genes (*ALG13*, *DNM1*, *GABRB3*, *HDAC4*) had de novo mutations in two or more probands. A follow-up study of *DNM1* done in collaboration with EuroEPINOMICS-Res provided further evidence that this gene was causative of epileptic encephalopathy.[22,37] Epi4K extended its investigations with a larger cohort of genetically unsolved cases of epileptic encephalopathy and reported evidence supporting *SLC1A2* and *CACNA1A* as disease etiologies in this syndrome.[38] In an additional case-control sequencing study conducted by Epi4K, the consortium demonstrated excess ultrarare variation in known epilepsy genes among persons with familial GGE, although no single gene was significantly associated with this syndrome.[39] Less enrichment was observed in sporadic non-acquired focal epilepsy. An exome sequencing study by CoGIE of EuroEPINOMICS identified variants in genes encoding GABA receptors among 152 families with GGE and validated the discovery in a second cohort of 357 sporadic cases.[40] These findings illustrated the power of exome sequencing to identify rare variants predisposing to epilepsy, and further illustrated that genes involved with rare familial epilepsy syndromes can also be associated with common forms of epilepsy.

The Epi4K Consortium also joined forces with a philanthropic foundation, Citizens United for Research in Epilepsy (CURE), to establish the Epilepsy Genetics Initiative (EGI). The primary purpose of the EGI was to reanalyze and reinterpret patient exome data periodically to identify genetic causes of epilepsy that may have been overlooked at the time of initial testing.[41,42] The initiative evaluated data from 166 probands and was successful in making 8 new diagnoses among 139 unsolved cases, a 5.8 percent yield. The findings emphasized the value of data sharing and collaboration in seeking a genetic diagnosis in epilepsy both in the research and clinical settings.

Another consortium (EpiPGX) was formed by investigators at 15 European institutions to identify genome-based biomarkers informative of individual responses to antiepileptic drugs. EpiPGX completed two studies examining the contribution of rare and common variants in determining the response to three commonly used drugs (valproic acid, levetiracetam, and lamotrigine).[43,44] The rare variant study was based on exome sequencing of 1,622 individuals treated with one of the three drugs, whereas a GWAS to examine common variants was conducted with 893 subjects. There were no common variants associated with drug response at a genome-wide significance level, likely because of limited study power. The exome study did demonstrate significant enrichment of rare variants among individuals resistant to valproic acid and levetiracetam, but only in subsets of genes with known involvement either in drug metabolism of valproic acid (*UGT1A3*, *UTG1A4*) or genes encoding synaptic vesicle glycoproteins (*SV2A*, *SV2B*), which are molecular targets of levetiracetam. Therefore, this study implicated genome-encoded variation in pharmacokinetics and pharmacodynamics of antiepileptic drugs as contributing to resistance to antiseizure medications, but there were no single gene variants with large effect sizes.

Epi4K was the inaugural NINDS-funded Center without Walls, but three more funding initiatives of this kind have promoted research in related areas. In 2014, NINDS funded the Center for SUDEP Research to study sudden unexplained death in epilepsy (SUDEP) comprising 12 principal investigators at 11 institutions across the United States and Europe with expertise in molecular biology, genetics, histopathology, electrophysiology, brain imaging, and data analysis. The Center included an emphasis on discovery of genetic factors that predispose to SUDEP in susceptible individuals. In 2016 and 2018, NINDS funded two additional Centers without Walls including the Epilepsy Bioinformatics Study for Antiepileptogenic Therapy to investigate post-traumatic epilepsy, and the Channelopathy-associated Epilepsy Research Center that investigates the functional consequences of genetic variants in epilepsy-associated ion channel genes. The creation of these research centers illustrates how funders can drive collaborative research in epilepsy.

Perhaps the most ambitious collaborative project in epilepsy genetics to date is Epi25, which aspires to sequence the exomes of 25,000 persons with epilepsy. The idea of Epi25 was born in 2014 at the Annual Meeting of the American Epilepsy Society and built upon the previous efforts by the ILAE Commission on Genetics, EuroEPINOMICS, and EPGP/Epi4K. This massive undertaking was accomplished by the sequencing center at the Broad Institute in Cambridge, Massachusetts with funding from NHGRI. The driving principle behind Epi25 is the power of collaboration to make more rapid progress toward understanding the genetic etiologies of epilepsy. An initial publication from this collaborative effort reported findings from exome sequencing of 9,170 epilepsy-affected individuals along with more than 8,000 controls. There was an excess of ultrarare, deleterious variants found in genes previously associated with epilepsy in individuals with epilepsy compared with controls, with the greatest enrichment in persons with developmental and epileptic encephalopathy. Cases of non-acquired focal epilepsy had the least enrichment. Variants in genes encoding GABA receptors and related pathways and voltage-gated cation channels were among the most significantly associated, but no single gene achieved exome-wide significance. These findings further underscore the contributions of rare genetic variation in the genesis of epilepsy. Beyond monogenic contributions to epilepsy, emerging scientific approaches are being applied to defining polygenic risk for epilepsy (see next section), and these efforts will similarly benefit from well-orchestrated collaborative networks including Epi25 to ensure sufficiently powered study populations.[45]

Genetic research in epilepsy can be catalyzed by efforts to aggregate clinical and genetic data together in an accessible format. This is illustrated by the Rational Intervention for KCNQ2/3 Epileptic Encephalopathy (RIKEE) Project. The mission of RIKEE is to provide access to comprehensive, curated information about known variants in two genes (*KCNQ2, KCNQ3*) responsible for a spectrum of early-onset epilepsy and epileptic encephalopathy. A database uniquely combines information on phenotype and functional consequences of individual variants that is valuable to researchers, clinicians, and families. Affiliations with parent-led organizations and funders enhance the impact of this resource.

The number of genes associated with monogenic epilepsy has exploded in recent years (Figure 2), and this evolution has driven diagnostic genetic testing to become standard of care in many situations. Out of this came a need to more formally adjudicate genes to ensure that their inclusion on a genetic test panel was clinically valid. This task was undertaken by the ClinGen Epilepsy Gene Curation Panel,[46] a group comprised of clinical epileptologists, medical geneticists, genetic counselors, clinical molecular geneticists, basic scientists, and biocurators, who use a framework established by the NIH-funded Clinical Genome Resource (ClinGen) that considers whether existing genetic and experimental evidence supports a true gene–disease association. The output of the curation panel is an expert classification of genes based on the level of evidence available with typical assessments of definitive, strong, limited, and disputed. In a pilot phase study, 16 genes were evaluated and classified. Eight genes received definitive or strong classifications (*ALG13, CHD2, DNM1, KCNQ2, KCNT1, SCN8A, STXBP1,* and *KCNA2*), while 3 genes were considered to have limited evidence supporting a gene–disease association (*GRIN2D, RYR3, SCN9A*). The final 5 genes were classified as disputed based on insufficient evidence (*CACNA1H, CACNB4, EFHC1, MAGI2, SRPX2*). The work of the panel will continue and findings will likely evolve as new evidence emerges. A long-term goal is to apply additional evidentiary classification rules to assess clinical validity of individual variants in the definitive genes.

Community groups and patient advocacy organizations have provided important drivers for collaboration among researchers. This has been accomplished by three means. Many organizations host annual or biennial family–professional conferences that bring together patients and their families with clinicians and researchers. These meetings provide a forum to educate families about current research endeavors and recent discoveries, and at the same time

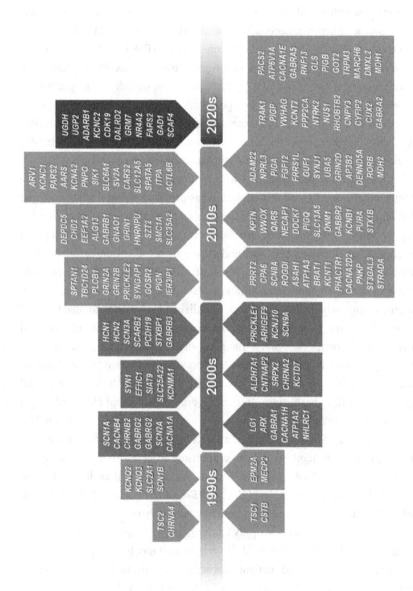

Figure 2 Timeline of epilepsy gene discoveries during the past 25 years.

provide opportunities for researchers to learn about the patient/family experience. Some groups also engage in raising funds for research and directly participate in studies seeking to illuminate the natural history of specific disorders.[47–50] Lastly, organic interactions with patients and families can motivate scientists in a manner distinct from the usual pursuits of academic success. Researchers motivated by altruism to help persons suffering with epilepsy often overcome concerns about competition, leading to greater sharing of knowledge and a stronger willingness to collaborate.

5 Advancing Gene Discovery in Epilepsy

Erin L. Heinzen, PharmD, PhD
University of North Carolina, Chapel Hill

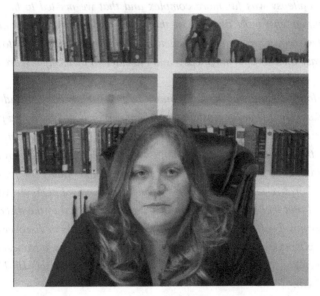

Video 5: Erin L. Heinzen, PharmD PhD. Video available at www.cambridge.org/poduri.

Video 5 transcript

[Erin Heinzen, PharmD PhD] Hello, everyone. I am Erin Heinzen. I'm an Associate Professor at the University of North Carolina in the Eshelman School of Pharmacy and the Department of Genetics in the School of Medicine. I have a Doctor of Pharmacy degree and also a PhD in pharmaceutical sciences.

For the last ten years or so, my research has focused on epilepsy genetics. While this might seem like an odd research focus for a pharmaceutical scientist, I am here because I believe the key to improved treatment of most neurological disorders lies in better understanding of the genetic underpinnings.

When I was in pharmacy school in the late 1990s, we were taught that epilepsy was largely a single-gene disorder. There were about 15–20 medications to treat seizures, but there was very little guidance on which medications would work best in the different types of seizures. This was in stark contrast to how cancer was presented to us, where there was much more consideration about the specific tumor types and also emerging ideas about targeted therapy.

While studying epilepsy pharmacogenomics during my postdoctoral training with Dr. David Goldstein at Duke University, it became clear that epilepsy was far more complex and that we needed to be thinking about epilepsy more like how we thought about cancer. It was at this point that we fully appreciated that genetics could provide a window into specific disease mechanisms in epilepsy, and I decided to focus my research efforts in this area.

Alongside many of the great minds in epilepsy genetics, including Sam Berkovic and Dan Lowenstein whom you met or heard from in a previous segment, and also my long-time mentor David Goldstein, we marched our way through genome-wide association studies, studies of rare copy number variation, early exome sequencing studies, and finally to large-scale collaborative sequencing work of Epi4K and now Epi25. As you have heard and will hear throughout this Element, this led to the discovery of many novel epilepsy genes. It took more than ten years to discover the first 20 epilepsy genes, and now – thanks in large part to advancements in sequencing technology – we are discovering on average 10–15 genes per year.

Despite this remarkable progress, only 10 percent of individuals with epilepsy have a clear genetic diagnosis. This suggests that there is much more to be found and that our search for epilepsy genes is far from complete. Like we were back in 2007, when next-generation sequencing first became available, I feel we are again at the precipice of many great discoveries that will be made possible through recent technological advancements.

In this section, I'll discuss the possible reasons why some epilepsy-causing genetic variants have yet to be identified and what the next steps are that will allow us to continue to drive forward gene discovery in epilepsy.

Over the last ten years, we have seen unprecedented advancements in our understanding of the genetic bases of epilepsy. Genome-wide genotyping and sequencing technologies facilitated the discovery of more than 100 genes or genomic loci involved in the risk of developing epilepsy. Identifying the types and origins of the risk alleles involved in these disorders has also allowed for our first glimpses at the underlying genetic architecture of epilepsy, including the following: (1) epilepsy is highly genetically heterogeneous; (2) many of the genes known to cause epilepsy encode proteins involved in neural transmission; (3) de novo (non-inherited) variants, including those exclusively present in the gametes of parents (parental mosaicism) and those arising post-zygotically, are important genetic contributors to epilepsy; (4) large genomic deletions, and particularly those overlapping copy number variant hotspots, contribute to a significant fraction of genetic risk of epilepsy; (5) many of the genes that underlie severe early-onset subtypes also carry variants that increase the risk for less severe subtypes.[36,39,51–53] This knowledge forms the foundation from which we can define the next phases of research into epilepsy genetics, to begin to explain the nearly 90 percent of individuals with epilepsy who remain genetically unexplained.

The driving force of technology

Technological advancements unquestionably drove recent progress in the understanding of the genetic underpinnings of epilepsy and many other diseases. Genome-wide genotyping arrays that use single nucleotide polymorphisms to tag common haplotypes defined by the HapMap Consortium provided us the first unbiased scans of the entire genome and pointed us early on to novel epilepsy risk loci in common forms of epilepsy. Microarray-based comparative array hybridization technologies, using small complementary DNA probes to scan for genomic gains or losses across the genome, revolutionized the ability to scan genome-wide copy number variants much smaller than possible with karyotyping and much more efficiently than possible with fluorescence in situ hybridization approaches.

Likewise, next-generation sequencing transformed our basic understanding of small genetic variants (single nucleotide substitution and small insertion or deletion variants) in the human population and helped geneticists to home in on small variants that were most likely to cause disease. This technology, historically referred to as massively parallel sequencing, works by performing parallel sequencing of amplified fragments of genomic DNA from the entire genome or select portions of the genome (i.e., whole exome or selected genes) to result in billions of sequenced copies of the original genomic DNA fragments. Each of these fragments is then aligned to the reference genome to result in a stack of reads covering each sequenced base. Once placed onto the reference genome, the reads can be scanned for alterations consistent with small genetic variants to reconstruct the unique DNA sequence from the individual. The true value of this technology was not only its deployment in genomic DNA from patients but also using it to establish the patterns of variation found across populations. By knowing what is normally present in the genome of individuals without a disease, scientists can better predict when a genetic variant might result in disease.

While we still are discovering genes rapidly with short-read exome sequencing (i.e., next-generation sequencing), the expectation is that soon the rate of gene discovery will plateau as we approach the point where we have learned all there is to learn from this technology. We now must look to new technological advancements that will take epilepsy genetics to the next level.

Transitioning from next- to third-generation sequencing

In principle, short-read next-generation sequencing would be able to sequence the entire genome, assuming that each sequenced DNA fragment is unique, all the pieces of the fragmented DNA can be sequenced with approximately equal efficiency and accuracy, the reference genome is precisely known at each of the 3 billion bases, and each fragment can be accurately associated with the chromosome of origin. However, the genome is far too complex with paralogs, homologs, genomic rearrangements, regions with high G-C content, and repetitive regions to achieve comprehensive whole-genome sequencing. While it is unlikely that we will achieve this ideal in the near future even with technological advancement, new long-read sequencing will get us a step closer by allowing us to better sequence complex regions of the human genome and to study genetic variants in the context of more-complete haplotypes (Figure 3).

Pacific BioSciences and Oxford Nanopore are the two "third-generation" long-read sequencing technologies that have the ability to sequence long DNA fragments (>100-fold longer than short-read technologies) without in vitro amplification of the DNA fragments prior to sequencing. Given the prominent role of rare, often de novo, protein-coding variants in epilepsy,[22,30,36] it is very likely that there are additional rare variant risk factors that could be readily detected with this new technology. Several recent reports have shown the utility of this technology in identifying pathogenic variations missed by short-read sequencing.[54–57]

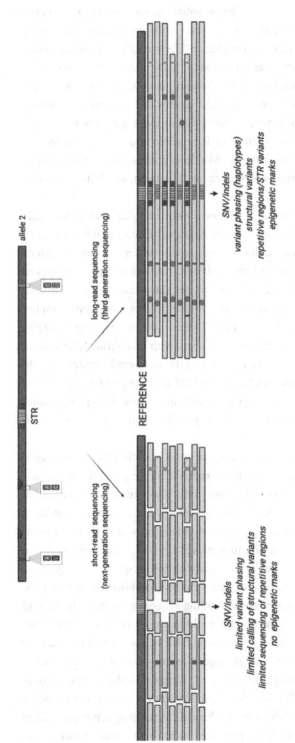

Figure 3 Comparison of variant calling potential of next- and third-generation sequencing technology.

Of particular note in epilepsy is the potential for long-read sequencing to capture short tandem repeat (STR) variation with much greater accuracy than possible with short-read sequencing. STRs are DNA sequences composed of sequentially repeated 1–6 base pair units. These repetitive sequences comprise ~3 percent of the human genome. Pathogenic expansions are uniquely found in neurological diseases and are prone to acquiring de novo sequence and length variants due to the highly mutable nature of the repetitive sequence,[58] making it possible and perhaps likely that they may also contribute to epilepsy. Multiple groups have already implicated intronic tandemly repeated sequences in a form of adult-onset myoclonic epilepsy.[59–63]

Beyond short tandem repeat variation, long-read sequencing will also offer an opportunity for higher-resolution scans of copy number variants. The association of genomic deletions and small variants (point mutations and small insertion-deletion variants) that result in loss of highly conserved proteins in epilepsy is clear,[22,30,64–66] but short-read NGS and microarray technologies are largely limited to identifying rare copy number variants greater than ~10 kb and indels less ~100 bps in length.[67,68] Additional epilepsy risk likely lies in this vast gap of intermediately sized genomic deletions and will be revealed with long-read sequencing. In addition, long-read sequencing has the added advantage of being able to sequence through complex structural variants and allow for typically more precise detection of breakpoints than possible with short-read next-generation sequencing.

Another likely source of yet-to-be-discovered genetic risk in epilepsy is rare variation in noncoding, regulatory regions of the genome. Such variation can be captured with whole-genome short-read next-generation sequencing, although it is challenging to interpret the impact of genetic variation on gene expression. Long-read sequencing will offer two advantages that will improve our ability to interpret noncoding sequencing. First, the new technology will allow for determining longer-range haplotypes to accurately assess compound heterozygous variant combinations that may be located both in and around the protein-coding sequence, without the need to sequence trios to establish phasing. Recently, unexpected second alleles for biallelic *ABCA4* disease have been found,[69] suggesting that recessive mechanisms may be playing a larger role than currently understood due to the challenges of identifying pathogenic variant pair combinations. Second, long-read sequencing will allow for haplotype rather than single variation association testing. One of the more striking findings in epilepsy genetics is that the same variant or variants predicted to have the same effect on the protein can have highly variable disease presentations. Such differences could be due to other variants in the gene that may modify phenotypes, as has been suggested by recent studies evaluating the effects of *cis*-acting regulatory variation on rare pathogenic variant penetrance.[70] If *cis*-acting modifiers do explain some fraction of pleiotropy in epilepsy, long-read sequencing would provide much greater opportunities to detect them.

The value of long-read sequencing can also be appreciated at the gene expression level. It is well accepted that the brain has higher rates of alternative splicing and novel brain-tissue-specific exons,[71,72] making annotation and interpretation of rare, noncanonical protein-coding variants found in diseases of the brain particularly challenging. Long-read RNA sequencing has been used to identify novel transcript isoforms caused by alternative splicing or novel exon usage,[73] which may be invaluable to the interpretation of intronic and other "noncoding" variation. This technology has recently been used to transcript isoform diversity for neuropsychiatric disease gene *CACNA1C*.[74]

Revealing the secrets of the single cell

In addition to long-read sequencing, advancements in single-cell sequencing technology now allow scientists to study pathophysiological processes at a resolution that has never before been possible. Single-cell DNA and RNA sequencing technologies allow for single-cell DNA sequencing and quantitative genome-wide assessments of the transcriptome at the single-cell level. These technologies have transformed our ability to study cellular lineages, identify rare cell types, identify gene expression regulatory networks in particular cell types, and explore how biological perturbations affect cell-type-specific gene expression. Given the unique availability of freshly resected tissue in some refractory epilepsy patients undergoing surgery, these single-cell technologies will likely offer novel insight into epileptogenic processes.

Most notable is the ability of this technology to more comprehensively explore the role of somatic variation in epilepsy. Post-zygotically acquired de novo mutations can arise at any point during development or throughout life to give rise to mosaicism. Depending on the timing of the mutational event, the cells harboring the genetic variant may be restricted to particular tissues or even individual cells. In the past ten years, there is increasing appreciation for the role of somatic variation in focal epilepsy that is typically associated with a focal cortical brain malformation. These pathogenic genetic variants are believed to arise during embryonic development. The majority of known pathogenic somatic variants were discovered through bulk tissue sequencing looking for heterozygous genetic variants that deviated from the expected 50 percent allelic presence and were confirmed with either single-cell or quantitative genotyping approaches. Most pathogenic somatic variants discovered to date reside in genes comprising the PI3 K-AKT-mTOR signaling pathway and lead to a constellation of phenotypes that are all associated with focal cortical dysplasia type II pathology.[51,52,75] Somatic variants in *SLC35A2*, encoding a UDP-galactose transporter, have been identified in the brain tissue radiographically non-lesional epilepsy patients with focal cortical dysplasia type I.[53,76] Interestingly, the clinical phenotypes of these mosaic epilepsy disorders appear to be related to the burden and likely the cell types harboring the pathogenic variants.[53,77] The application of single-cell genomic technologies will greatly improve our ability to identify post-zygotically acquired de novo variants in epilepsy and will provide a unique lens for elucidating the role of different cell types involved in epileptogenesis.

Polygenic risk in epilepsy

While the vast majority of epilepsy risk loci identified to date are rare and very highly penetrant, it is very likely that combinations of genetic variants across the allelic frequency spectrum also contribute to disease risk. Polygenic risk, as assessed through common variant signal, is already reproducibly detectable across multiple types of epilepsy.[45] In addition, there are an increasing number of examples where variants predicted to have the same effect on the gene result in highly variable phenotypes. With increasingly large cohorts of epilepsy patients being exome sequenced through collaborative initiatives like Epi25 and in-depth analyses of multiplex epilepsy families with variable presentations, polygenic risk factors will likely emerge as significant contributors of unexplained epilepsy risk and pleiotropy.

Overview

As we did during the early phases of short-read next-generation sequencing, the research community will face challenges initially to readily perform long-read and single-cell RNA sequencing due to the expense and the technical and analysis hurdles associated with any new genomic technology. However, the potential for the technology to take disease genetics, including epilepsy, to the next level is clear. We can be comforted by our prior experience of seeing how technology can rapidly evolve to drive essential research forward even further toward pathophysiological insights and novel pharmacological targets.

Glossary

Allele – a variant or version of a gene that may produce a variation in a trait (example, eye color).

Array – a tool that allows placement of DNA fragments on probes where they can be quantified and the sequence at a particular site determined.

Channelopathy – a disorder caused by disturbed structure or function of ion channels, which regulate neural signals in the body.

Copy number – within a genome, the number of copies of a specific fragment of DNA.

Copy number variant – regions of DNA that are either partially or completely deleted (missing) or duplicated (present in excess amount).

de novo – newly arising; for example, a de novo variant as opposed to an inherited variant.

Electrophysiology – study of the electrical functions, for example, of the brain or heart.

Epidemiology – study of where, why, and in whom disease or other health events occur.

Epilepsy – condition defined by more than one unprovoked seizure (also used when a person has a single seizure in the setting of risk factors for recurrence that result in the initiation of an anti-seizure medication).

Epileptic encephalopathy – early-onset epilepsy in which the electrophysiological abnormalities present and/or seizures are thought to contribute to brain dysfunction.

Epileptogenesis – the processes that lead to the development of epilepsy.

Etiology – the cause of a disease or disorder.

Exome – part of the genome. The exome is made of up exons, the coding portion of DNA.

Exon – DNA sequence that encodes for amino acids (building blocks of protein).

Gamete – a reproductive cell; contains one set of chromosomes.

Gene – the functional unit of heredity; a sequence of nucleotides on a chromosome that determines a trait.

Genome – all genetic material within an organism including, for example, DNA, RNA, and mitochondrial DNA.

Genome-wide association study (GWAS) – a study that seeks to identify single nucleotide polymorphisms in individuals with versus without a disease.

Genomics – the study of the genome.

Genotype – (noun) the genetic makeup of an organism. (verb) to determine an organism's genetic makeup.

Germ cell – cells that produce gametes through meiosis.

Haplotype – closely linked DNA sequences usually inherited together from a single chromosome.

Histopathology – the study of tissue changes seen in disease.

Inheritance – the passage of genetic material from parents to offspring.

Autosomal dominant inheritance – refers to a disease or trait inherited through a single copy of a gene.

Autosomal recessive inheritance – refers to a disease inherited through two copies of a gene, one from each parent.

Oligogenic inheritance – refers to a disease or trait influenced by a small number of genes.

X-linked inheritance – refers to a disease or trait inherited from one parent, where the gene is located on the X chromosome.

Intron – noncoding DNA sequence between exons.

Linkage analysis – statistical correlation of data regarding a specific gene in order to identify its location on the chromosome.

Locus (plural "loci") – location or site.

Locus heterogeneity – variants in different genes causing similar syndromes.

Meiosis – the process by which germ cells divide to produce gametes.

Microdeletion – a change in a chromosome wherein a small piece of the chromosome is removed.

Monogenic – arising from one gene.

Mosaicism – genetic mosaicism is the presence of cells with different genetic profiles intermixed in the same organism or tissue; in the context of epilepsy genetics, mosaic variants arise through post-zygotic mutational events occurring at varying times during development and result in a mixture of variant-positive and variant-negative cells.

Parental (gamete, or gonadal) mosaicism – mosaicism affecting egg and sperm of parents.

Mutation – an event that results in a change in the DNA composition or quantity, often but not restricted to the time when one cell divides to produce two cells.

Nucleotide – a molecular organic compound; when nucleotides link together, they form the basis of DNA and RNA.

Pathogenic – able to cause disease.

Pharmacodynamics – the relationship between concentration of a drug at its site of action and the resulting effects.

Pharmacokinetics – how the body absorbs, distributes, metabolizes, and eliminates a drug.

Phenotype – (noun) the combined appearance of traits or characteristics in an organism or subgroup. (verb) to perform comparative analyses to discover common traits or characteristics. (adjective "phenotyped") describes subjects grouped by analysis into a phenotype.

Polygenic – arising from more than one gene.

Precision medicine – the use of genetic findings to personalize medical treatments.

Proband – a subject who is being studied.

Seizure – abnormal and organized rhythmic electrical activity that may or may not result in an outward clinical manifestation.

Sequencing – a process that identifies the arrangement of individual nucleotides within a molecule of DNA.

Long-read sequencing – also known as "third-generation sequencing"; NGS of longer sequencing fragments that allows for better sequencing of complex regions in the genome.

Next-generation sequencing (NGS) – also known as "short-read exome sequencing" or "massively parallel sequencing." Short DNA fragments are sequenced in parallel and reassembled on the genome to determine the genomic sequence of the targeted regions.

Single-cell sequencing – NGS of DNA or RNA from individual cells.

Whole exome sequencing (WES) – sequencing of the entire protein-coding area (exome) of a genome.

Whole genome sequencing (WGS) – sequencing of the protein-coding (exome) and noncoding areas of a genome.

Single nucleotide polymorphism – a variation in a small area of the genome.

Somatic cells – cells that are not involved in reproduction but in the composition of the body.

Sudden unexplained death in epilepsy (SUDEP) – a major cause of death in patients with epilepsy, when the death of an otherwise healthy person with epilepsy is not related to trauma or other found cause.

Translational research – a process of research aimed toward translating laboratory findings into clinical practice.

Twins, monozygotic/dizygotic – monozygotic or "identical" twins develop from a single fertilized egg. Dizygotic or "fraternal" twins develop from two different fertilized eggs.

Variant – a genetic change, resulting from a mutational event, that can be detected in the form of a single nucleotide change, copy number loss (deletion) or gain (duplication), or structural rearrangement (e.g., chromosomal inversion).

Germline variant – a genetic change within germ cells.

Short tandem repeat (STR) variation –   a genetic change in a DNA sequence composed of sequentially repeated 1–6 base pair units.

Somatic mosaic variant – a genetic change present in some but not all cells in a particular tissue, resulting from mutation occurring after the one-cell developmental stage.

Variant expressivity – a single mutation in one gene resulting in different syndromes.

Zygote – a fertilized egg prior to its subdivision into multiple cells.

References

1. O. Temkin, *The Falling Sickness* (Baltimore MD: The Johns Hopkins Press; 1945).
2. J. R. Reynolds, *Epilepsy: Its Symptoms, Treatment, and Relation to Other Chronic Convulsive Diseases* (John Churchill; 1861).
3. F. Leuret, Recherches sur l'epilepsie, *Archives Generales de Medecine*, 4th series, 2 (1843), 32–50.
4. W. G. Lennox, M. A. Lennox, The Genetics of Epilepsy. *Epilepsy and Related Disorders*, vol. 1 (Boston MA: Little, Brown; 1960), pp. 532–74.
5. J. F. Annegers, W. A. Hauser, L. R. Elveback, V. E. Anderson, L. I. Kurland, Congenital malformations and seizure disorders in the offspring of parents with epilepsy, *Int J Epidemiol*, 7 (1978), 241–7. DOI: https://doi.org/10.1093/ije/7.3.241.
6. J. F. Annegers, W. A. Hauser, V. E. Anderson, L. T. Kurland, The risks of seizure disorders among relatives of patients with childhood onset epilepsy, *Neurology*, 32 (1982), 174–9. DOI: https://doi.org/10.1212/wnl.32.2.174.
7. M. Leppert, V. E. Anderson, T. Quattlebaum, D. Stauffer, P. O'Connell, Y. Nakamura, et al., Benign familial neonatal convulsions linked to genetic markers on chromosome 20, *Nature*, 337 (1989), 647–8. DOI: https://doi.org/10.1038/337647a0.
8. C. Biervert, B. C. Schroeder, C. Kubisch, S. F. Berkovic, P. Propping, T. J. Jentsch, et al., A potassium channel mutation in neonatal human epilepsy, *Science*, 279 (1998), 403–6. DOI: https://doi.org/10.1126/science.279.5349.403.
9. O. K. Steinlein, J. C. Mulley, P. Propping, R. H. Wallace, H. A. Phillips, G. R. Sutherland, et al., A missense mutation in the neuronal nicotinic acetylcholine receptor alpha 4 subunit is associated with autosomal dominant nocturnal frontal lobe epilepsy, *Nat Genet*, 11 (1995), 201–3. DOI: https://doi.org/10.1038/ng1095-201.
10. EPICURE Consortium, EMINet Consortium, M. Steffens, C. Leu, A. K. Ruppert, F. Zara, et al., Genome-wide association analysis of genetic generalized epilepsies implicates susceptibility loci at 1q43, 2p16.1, 2q22.3 and 17q21.32, *Hum Mol Genet*, 21 (2012), 5359–72. DOI: https://doi.org/10.1093/hmg/dds373.
11. International Human Genome Sequencing Consortium, Finishing the euchromatic sequence of the human genome, *Nature*, 431 (2004), 931–45. DOI: https://doi.org/10.1038/nature03001.

12. International HapMap Consortium, The International HapMap Project, *Nature*, 426 (2003), 789–96. DOI: https://doi.org/10.1038/nature02168.

13. 1000 Genomes Project Consortium, A. Auton, L. D. Brooks, R. M. Durbin, E. P. Garrison, H. M. Kang, et al., A global reference for human genetic variation, *Nature*, 526 (2015), 68–74. DOI: https://doi.org/10.1038/nature15393.

14. A. E. Fryer, A. Chalmers, J. M. Connor, I. Fraser, S. Povey, A. D. Yates, et al., Evidence that the gene for tuberous sclerosis is on chromosome 9, *Lancet*, 1 (1987), 659–61. DOI: https://doi.org/10.1016/s0140-6736(87)90416-8.

15. R. S. Kandt, J. L. Haines, M. Smith, H. Northrup, R. J. Gardner, M. P. Short, et al., Linkage of an important gene locus for tuberous sclerosis to a chromosome 16 marker for polycystic kidney disease, *Nat Genet*, 2 (1992), 37–41. DOI: https://10.1038/ng0992-37.

16. European Chromosome 16 Tuberous Sclerosis Consortium, Identification and characterization of the tuberous sclerosis gene on chromosome 16, *Cell*, 75 (1993), 1305–15. DOI: https://doi.org/10.1016/0092-8674(93)90618-z.

17. M. van Slegtenhorst, R. de Hoogt, C. Hermans, M. Nellist, B. Janssen, S. Verhoef, et al., Identification of the tuberous sclerosis gene TSC1 on chromosome 9q34, *Science*, 277 (1997), 805–8. DOI: https://doi.org/10.1126/science.277.5327.805.

18. EPICURE Consortium, C. Leu, C. G. de Kovel, F. Zara, P. Striano, M. Pezzella, et al., Genome-wide linkage meta-analysis identifies susceptibility loci at 2q34 and 13q31.3 for genetic generalized epilepsies, *Epilepsia*, 53 (2012), 308–18. DOI: https://doi.org/10.1111/j.1528-1167.2011.03379.x.

19. International League Against Epilepsy Consortium on Complex Epilepsies, Genetic determinants of common epilepsies: a meta-analysis of genome-wide association studies, *Lancet Neurol*, 13 (2014), 893–903. DOI: https://doi.org/10.1016/S1474-4422(14)70171-1.

20. International League Against Epilepsy Consortium on Complex Epilepsies, Genome-wide mega-analysis identifies 16 loci and highlights diverse biological mechanisms in the common epilepsies, *Nat Commun*, 9 (2018), 5269. DOI: https://doi.org/10.1038/s41467-018-07524-z.

21. G. L. Carvill, J. M. McMahon, A. Schneider, M. Zemel, C. T. Myers, J. Saykally, et al., Mutations in the GABA transporter SLC6A1 cause epilepsy with myoclonic-atonic seizures, *Am J Hum Genet*, 96 (2015), 808–15. DOI: https://doi.org/10.1016/j.ajhg.2015.02.016.

22. Euro-EPINOMICS-RES Consortium, Epilepsy Phenome/Genome Project, Epi4K Consortium, De novo mutations in synaptic transmission genes including DNM1 cause epileptic encephalopathies, *Am J Hum Genet*, 95 (2014), 360–70. DOI: https://doi.org/10.1016/j.ajhg.2014.08.013.

23. C. Nava, C. Dalle, A. Rastetter, P. Striano, C. G. de Kovel, R. Nabbout, et al., De novo mutations in HCN1 cause early infantile epileptic encephalopathy, *Nat Genet*, 46 (2014), 640–5. DOI: https://doi.org/10.1038/ng.2952.

24. J. Schubert, A. Siekierska, M. Langlois, P. May, C. Huneau, F. Becker, et al., Mutations in STX1B, encoding a presynaptic protein, cause fever-associated epilepsy syndromes, *Nat Genet*, 46 (2014), 1327–32. DOI: https://doi.org/10.1038/ng.3130.

25. A. Suls, J. A. Jaehn, A. Kecskes, Y. Weber, S. Weckhuysen, D. C. Craiu, et al., De novo loss-of-function mutations in CHD2 cause a fever-sensitive myoclonic epileptic encephalopathy sharing features with Dravet syndrome, *Am J Hum Genet*, 93 (2013), 967–75. DOI: https://doi.org/10.1016/j.ajhg.2013.09.017.

26. S. Syrbe, U. B. S. Hedrich, E. Riesch, T. Djemie, S. Muller, R. S. Moller, et al., De novo loss- or gain-of-function mutations in KCNA2 cause epileptic encephalopathy, *Nat Genet*, 47 (2015), 393–9. DOI: https://doi.org/10.1038/ng.3239.

27. S. Tang, L. Addis, A. Smith, S. D. Topp, M. Pendziwiat, D. Mei, et al., Phenotypic and genetic spectrum of epilepsy with myoclonic atonic seizures, *Epilepsia*, 61 (2020), 995–1007. DOI: https://doi.org/10.1111/epi.16508.

28. J. Larsen, G. L. Carvill, E. Gardella, G. Kluger, G. Schmiedel, N. Barisic, et al., The phenotypic spectrum of SCN8A encephalopathy, *Neurology*, 84 (2015), 480–9. DOI: https://doi.org/10.1212/WNL.0000000000001211.

29. D. Lal, S. Steinbrucker, J. Schubert, T. Sander, F. Becker, Y. Weber, et al., Investigation of GRIN2A in common epilepsy phenotypes, *Epilepsy Res*, 115 (2015), 95–9. DOI: https://doi.org/10.1016/j.eplepsyres.2015.05.010.

30. H. O. Heyne, T. Singh, H. Stamberger, R. Abou Jamra, H. Caglayan, D. Craiu, et al., De novo variants in neurodevelopmental disorders with epilepsy, *Nat Genet*, 50 (2018), 1048–53. DOI: https://doi.org/10.1038/s41588-018-0143-7.

31. C. Marini, A. Porro, A. Rastetter, C. Dalle, I. Rivolta, D. Bauer, et al., HCN1 mutation spectrum: from neonatal epileptic encephalopathy to benign generalized epilepsy and beyond, *Brain*, 141 (2018), 3160–78. DOI: https://doi.org/10.1093/brain/awy263.

32. C. Mignot, C. von Stulpnagel, C. Nava, D. Ville, D. Sanlaville, G. Lesca, et al., Genetic and neurodevelopmental spectrum of SYNGAP1-associated intellectual disability and epilepsy, *J Med Genet*, 53 (2016), 511–22. DOI: https://doi.org/10.1136/jmedgenet-2015-103451.

33. EPGP Collaborative, B. Abou-Khalil, B. Alldredge, J. Bautista, S. Berkovic, J. Bluvstein, et al., The epilepsy phenome/genome project, *Clin Trials*, 10 (2013), 568–86. DOI: https://doi.org/10.1177/1740774513484392.

34. K. McGovern, C. F. Karn, K. Fox, E. Investigators, surpassing the target: how a recruitment campaign transformed the participant accrual trajectory in the Epilepsy Phenome/Genome Project, *Clin Transl Sci*, 8 (2015), 518–25. DOI: https://doi.org/10.1111/cts.12307.

35. Epi4K Consortium, Epi4K: gene discovery in 4,000 genomes, *Epilepsia*, 53 (2012), 1457–67. DOI: https://doi.org/10.1111/j.1528-1167.2012.03511.x.

36. Epi4K Consortium, Epilepsy Phenome/Genome Project, A. S. Allen, S. F. Berkovic, P. Cossette, N. Delanty, et al., De novo mutations in epileptic encephalopathies, *Nature*, 501 (2013), 217–21. DOI: https://doi.org/10.1038/nature12439.

37. S. von Spiczak, K. L. Helbig, D. N. Shinde, R. Huether, M. Pendziwiat, C. Lourenco, et al., DNM1 encephalopathy: A new disease of vesicle fission, *Neurology*, 89 (2017), 385–94. DOI: https://doi.org/10.1212/WNL.0000000000004152.

38. Epi4K Consortium, De novo mutations in SLC1A2 and CACNA1A are important causes of epileptic encephalopathies, *Am J Hum Genet*, 99 (2016), 287–98. DOI: https://doi.org/10.1016/j.ajhg.2016.06.003.

39. Epi4K Consortium, Epilepsy Phenome/Genome Project, Ultra-rare genetic variation in common epilepsies: a case-control sequencing study, *Lancet Neurol*, 16 (2017), 135–43. DOI: https://doi.org/10.1016/S1474-4422(16)30359-3.

40. P. May, S. Girard, M. Harrer, D. R. Bobbili, J. Schubert, S. Wolking, et al., Rare coding variants in genes encoding GABAA receptors in genetic generalised epilepsies: an exome-based case-control study, *Lancet Neurol*, 17 (2018), 699–708. DOI: https://doi.org/10.1016/S1474-4422(18)30215-1.

41. Epilepsy Genetics Initiative , De novo variants in the alternative exon 5 of SCN8A cause epileptic encephalopathy, *Genet Med*, 20 (2018), 275–81. DOI: https://doi.org/10.1038/gim.2017.100.

42. Epilepsy Genetics Initiative, The Epilepsy Genetics Initiative: Systematic reanalysis of diagnostic exomes increases yield, *Epilepsia*, 60 (2019), 797–806. DOI: https://doi.org/10.1111/epi.14698.

43. S. Wolking, C. Moreau, A. T. Nies, E. Schaeffeler, M. McCormack, P. Auce, et al., Testing association of rare genetic variants with resistance to three common antiseizure medications, *Epilepsia*, 61 (2020), 657–66. DOI: https://doi.org/10.1111/epi.16467.

44. S. Wolking, H. Schulz, A. T. Nies, M. McCormack, E. Schaeffeler, P. Auce, et al., Pharmacoresponse in genetic generalized epilepsy: a genome-wide association study, *Pharmacogenomics*, 21 (2020), 325–35. DOI: https://doi.org/10.2217/pgs-2019-0179.

45. C. Leu, R. Stevelink, A. W. Smith, S. B. Goleva, M. Kanai, L. Ferguson, et al., Polygenic burden in focal and generalized epilepsies, *Brain*, 142 (2019), 3473–81. DOI: https://doi.org/10.1093/brain/awz292.

46. I. Helbig, E. R. Riggs, C. A. Barry, K. M. Klein, D. Dyment, C. Thaxton, et al., The ClinGen Epilepsy Gene Curation Expert Panel – Bridging the divide between clinical domain knowledge and formal gene curation criteria, *Hum Mutat*, 39 (2018), 1476–84. DOI: https://doi.org/10.1002/humu.23632.

47. D. R. M. Vlaskamp, B. J. Shaw, R. Burgess, D. Mei, M. Montomoli, H. Xie, et al., SYNGAP1 encephalopathy: A distinctive generalized developmental and epileptic encephalopathy, *Neurology*, 92 (2019), e96-e107. DOI: https://doi.org/10.1212/WNL.0000000000006729.

48. A. T. Berg, S. Mahida, A. Poduri, KCNQ2-DEE: developmental or epileptic encephalopathy?, *Ann Clin Transl Neurol*, 8 (2021), 666–76. DOI: https://doi.org/10.1002/acn3.51316.

49. A. T. Berg, H. Palac, G. Wilkening, F. Zelko, L. Schust Meyer, SCN2A-Developmental and Epileptic Encephalopathies: Challenges to trial-readiness for non-seizure outcomes, *Epilepsia*, 62 (2021), 258–68. DOI: https://doi.org/10.1111/epi.16750.

50. A. Jimenez-Gomez, S. Niu, F. Andujar-Perez, E. A. McQuade, A. Balasa, D. Huss, et al., Phenotypic characterization of individuals with SYNGAP1 pathogenic variants reveals a potential correlation between posterior dominant rhythm and developmental progression, *J Neurodev Disord*, 11 (2019), 18. DOI: https://doi.org/10.1186/s11689-019-9276-y.

51. J. H. Lee, M. Huynh, J. L. Silhavy, S. Kim, T. Dixon-Salazar, A. Heiberg, et al., De novo somatic mutations in components of the PI3K-AKT3-mTOR pathway cause hemimegalencephaly, *Nat Genet*, 44 (2012), 941–5. DOI: https://doi.org/10.1038/ng.2329.

52. A. Poduri, G. D. Evrony, X. Cai, P. C. Elhosary, R. Beroukhim, M. K. Lehtinen, et al., Somatic activation of AKT3 causes hemispheric developmental brain malformations, *Neuron*, 74 (2012), 41–8. DOI: https://doi.org/10.1016/j.neuron.2012.03.010.

53. M. R. Winawer, N. G. Griffin, J. Samanamud, E. H. Baugh, D. Rathakrishnan, S. Ramalingam, et al., Somatic SLC35A2 variants in the brain are associated with intractable neocortical epilepsy, *Ann Neurol*, 83 (2018), 1133–46. DOI: https://doi.org/10.1002/ana.25243.

54. E. W. Loomis, J. S. Eid, P. Peluso, J. Yin, L. Hickey, D. Rank, et al., Sequencing the unsequenceable: expanded CGG-repeat alleles of the fragile X gene, *Genome Res*, 23 (2013), 121–8. DOI: https://doi.org/10.1101/gr.141705.112.

55. J. D. Merker, A. M. Wenger, T. Sneddon, M. Grove, Z. Zappala, L. Fresard, et al., Long-read genome sequencing identifies causal structural variation in a Mendelian disease, *Genet Med*, 20 (2018), 159–63. DOI: https://doi.org/10.1038/gim.2017.86.

56. A. Sanchis-Juan, J. Stephens, C. E. French, N. Gleadall, K. Megy, C. Penkett, et al., Complex structural variants in Mendelian disorders: identification and breakpoint resolution using short- and long-read genome sequencing, *Genome Med*, 10 (2018), 95. DOI: https://doi.org/10.1186/s13073-018-0606-6.

57. J. Sone, S. Mitsuhashi, A. Fujita, T. Mizuguchi, K. Hamanaka, K. Mori, et al., Long-read sequencing identifies GGC repeat expansions in NOTCH2NLC associated with neuronal intranuclear inclusion disease, *Nat Genet*, 51 (2019), 1215–21. DOI: https://doi.org/10.1038/s41588-019-0459-y.

58. H. Fan, J. Y. Chu, A brief review of short tandem repeat mutation, *Genomics Proteomics Bioinformatics*, 5 (2007), 7–14. DOI: https://doi.org/10.1016/S1672-0229(07)60009-6.

59. Z. Cen, Z. Jiang, Y. Chen, X. Zheng, F. Xie, X. Yang, et al., Intronic pentanucleotide TTTCA repeat insertion in the SAMD12 gene causes familial cortical myoclonic tremor with epilepsy type 1, *Brain*, 141 (2018), 2280–8. DOI: https://doi.org/10.1093/brain/awy160.

60. M. A. Corbett, T. Kroes, L. Veneziano, M. F. Bennett, R. Florian, A. L. Schneider, et al., Intronic ATTTC repeat expansions in STARD7 in familial adult myoclonic epilepsy linked to chromosome 2, *Nat Commun*, 10 (2019), 4920. DOI: https://doi.org/10.1038/s41467-019-12671-y.

61. R. T. Florian, F. Kraft, E. Leitao, S. Kaya, S. Klebe, E. Magnin, et al., Unstable TTTTA/TTTCA expansions in MARCH6 are associated with Familial Adult Myoclonic Epilepsy type 3, *Nat Commun*, 10 (2019), 4919. DOI: https://doi.org/10.1038/s41467-019-12763-9.

62. H. Ishiura, K. Doi, J. Mitsui, J. Yoshimura, M. K. Matsukawa, A. Fujiyama, et al., Expansions of intronic TTTCA and TTTTA repeats in benign adult

familial myoclonic epilepsy, *Nat Genet*, 50 (2018), 581–90. DOI: https://doi.org/10.1038/s41588-018-0067-2.

63. T. Mizuguchi, T. Toyota, H. Adachi, N. Miyake, N. Matsumoto, S. Miyatake, Detecting a long insertion variant in SAMD12 by SMRT sequencing: implications of long-read whole-genome sequencing for repeat expansion diseases, *J Hum Genet*, 64 (2019), 191–7. DOI: https://doi.org/10.1038/s10038-018-0551-7.

64. L. M. Niestroj, E. Perez-Palma, D. P. Howrigan, Y. Zhou, F. Cheng, E. Saarentaus, et al., Epilepsy subtype-specific copy number burden observed in a genome-wide study of 17 458 subjects, *Brain*, 143 (2020), 2106–18. DOI: https://doi.org/10.1093/brain/awaa171.

65. Epilepsy Phenome/Genome Project, Epi4K Consortium, Copy number variant analysis from exome data in 349 patients with epileptic encephalopathy, *Ann Neurol*, 78 (2015), 323–8. DOI: https://doi.org/10.1002/ana.24457.

66. Epi25 Collaborative, Ultra-rare genetic variation in the epilepsies: a whole-exome sequencing study of 17,606 individuals, *Am J Hum Genet*, 105 (2019), 267–82. DOI: https://doi.org/10.1016/j.ajhg.2019.05.020.

67. L. Zhang, W. Bai, N. Yuan, Z. Du, Comprehensively benchmarking applications for detecting copy number variation, *PLoS Comput Biol*, 15 (2019), e1007069. DOI: https://doi.org/10.1371/journal.pcbi.1007069.

68. B. P. Coe, B. Ylstra, B. Carvalho, G. A. Meijer, C. Macaulay, W. L. Lam , Resolving the resolution of array CGH, *Genomics*, 89 (2007), 647–53. DOI: https://doi.org/10.1016/j.ygeno.2006.12.012.

69. J. Zernant, W. Lee, F. T. Collison, G. A. Fishman, Y. V. Sergeev, K. Schuerch, et al., Frequent hypomorphic alleles account for a significant fraction of ABCA4 disease and distinguish it from age-related macular degeneration, *J Med Genet*, 54 (2017), 404–12. DOI: https://doi.org/10.1136/jmedgenet-2017-104540.

70. S. E. Castel, A. Cervera, P. Mohammadi, F. Aguet, F. Reverter, A. Wolman, et al., Modified penetrance of coding variants by cis-regulatory variation contributes to disease risk, *Nat Genet*, 50 (2018), 1327–34. DOI: https://doi.org/10.1038/s41588-018-0192-y.

71. B. Raj, B. J. Blencowe, Alternative splicing in the mammalian nervous system: recent insights into mechanisms and functional roles, *Neuron*, 87 (2015), 14–27. DOI: https://doi.org/10.1016/j.neuron.2015.05.004.

72. M. Mele, P. G. Ferreira, F. Reverter, D. S. DeLuca, J. Monlong, M. Sammeth, et al., Human genomics. The human transcriptome across tissues and individuals, *Science*, 348 (2015), 660–5. DOI: https://doi.org/10.1126/science.aaa0355.

73. P. Uapinyoying, J. Goecks, S. M. Knoblach, K. Panchapakesan, C. G. Bonnemann, T. A. Partridge, et al., A new long-read RNA-seq analysis approach identifies and quantifies novel transcripts of very large genes, *bioRxiv*, 01.08.898627 (2020). DOI: https://doi.org/doi.org/10.1101/2020.01.08.898627.

74. M. B. Clark, T. Wrzesinski, A. B. Garcia, N. A. L. Hall, J. E. Kleinman, T. Hyde, et al., Long-read sequencing reveals the complex splicing profile of the psychiatric risk gene CACNA1C in human brain, *Mol Psychiatry*, 25 (2020), 37–47. DOI: https://10.1038/s41380-019-0583-1.

75. J. S. Lim, R. Gopalappa, S. H. Kim, S. Ramakrishna, M. Lee, W. I. Kim, et al., Somatic mutations in TSC1 and TSC2 cause focal cortical dysplasia, *Am J Hum Genet*, 100 (2017), 454–72. DOI: https://doi.org/10.1016/j.ajhg.2017.01.030.

76. N. S. Sim, Y. Seo, J. S. Lim, W. K. Kim, H. Son, H. D. Kim, et al., Brain somatic mutations in SLC35A2 cause intractable epilepsy with aberrant N-glycosylation, *Neurol Genet*, 4 (2018), e294. DOI: https://doi.org/10.1212/NXG.0000000000000294.

77. A. M. D'Gama, M. B. Woodworth, A. A. Hossain, S. Bizzotto, N. E. Hatem, C. M. LaCoursiere, et al., Somatic mutations activating the mTOR pathway in dorsal telencephalic progenitors cause a continuum of cortical dysplasias, *Cell Rep*, 21 (2017), 3754–66. DOI: https://doi.org/10.1016/j.celrep.2017.11.106.

Cambridge Elements ☰

Genetics in Epilepsy

Lead Editor

Annapurna H. Poduri

Boston Children's Hospital, Harvard Medical School

Annapurna H. Poduri, MD, MPH is Professor of Neurology at Harvard Medical School. She is also Director of the Epilepsy Genetics Program at Boston Children's Hospital, which focuses on the discovery of germline and mosaic variants in patients with epilepsy, and modeling epilepsy genes in zebrafish and cell-based models.

Deputy Editors

Alfred L. George, Jr.

Northwestern University Feinberg School of Medicine

Alfred L. George, Jr., MD is Professor and Chair of Pharmacology at the Northwestern University Feinberg School of Medicine. He directs the Channelopathy-associated Epilepsy Research Center without Walls, supported by the National Institutes of Neurological Disorders and Stroke, connecting patient variants with bench science.

Erin L. Heinzen

University of North Carolina, Chapel Hill

Erin L. Heinzen, PharmD, PhD is Associate Professor of Pharmacy and Genetics at the University of North Carolina at Chapel Hill. She has served as Principal Investigator of the Sequencing, Biostatistics & Bioinformatics Core of the Epi4K Consortium and investigates somatic mosaic mutation in epilepsy and the mechanisms underlying SLC35A2 epilepsy.

Daniel Lowenstein

University of California, San Francisco

Daniel Lowenstein, MD is Professor of Neurology at the University of California, San Francisco. He has served as Principal Investigator of the Epilepsy Phenome/Genome Project and the Epi4K Consortium, is active in many international collaborative initiatives, and is past chair of the Genetics Commission of the International League Against Epilepsy.

Associate Editor

Sara James

Journalist and author

Sara James is a renowned broadcast journalist and an advocate for research in epilepsy and community-academic partnerships in genetic epilepsy. She is Vice President of the KCNQ2 Cure Alliance and a co-founder of Genetic Epilepsy Team Australia.

About the Series

Recent advances in epilepsy genetics are actively revealing numerous genetic contributors to epilepsy, both inherited and non-inherited, collectively accounting for a substantial portion of otherwise unexplained epilepsies. This series integrates clinical epilepsy genetics and laboratory research, driving the field towards more precise and effective treatments.

Printed in the United States
by Baker & Taylor Publisher Services